natural
SEX
BOOSTERS

Supplements that Enhance Stamina, Sensation, and Sexuality for Men and Women

Ray Sahelian, MD

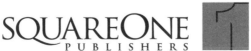

SQUAREONE
PUBLISHERS

The information and advice contained in this book are based upon the research and the personal and professional experiences of the author. They are not intended as a substitute for consulting with a health care professional. The publisher and author are not responsible for any adverse effects or consequences resulting from the use of any of the suggestions, preparations, or procedures discussed in this book. All matters pertaining to your physical health should be supervised by a health care professional. It is a sign of wisdom, not cowardice, to seek a second or third opinion.

COVER DESIGNER: Phaedra Mastrocola
COVER PHOTO: Getty Images, Inc.
IN-HOUSE EDITOR: Elaine Kennedy
TYPESETTER: Gary A. Rosenberg

Square One Publishers
115 Herricks Road
Garden City Park, NY 11040
(516) 535-2010 • (877) 900-BOOK
www.squareonepublishers.com

Publisher's Cataloging-in-Publication Data
Sahelian, Ray.
    Natural sex boosters : supplements that enhance stamina,
sensation, and sexuality for men and women / Ray Sahelian.
        p. cm.
    Includes bibliographical references and index.
    ISBN 978-0-7570-0141-3
    1. Aphrodisiacs. 2. Dietary supplements. 3. Sexual disorders—
Alternative treatment. I. Title.
RM386.S34 2004
615'.766—dc22

                                         2004000598

Printed in Canada

10   9   8   7   6   5   4   3   2

Contents

Introduction: Understanding the Human Sexual Response, 1

1. Sex Chemistry Made Simple, 13

2. Androstenedione: The Father of Testosterone, 19

3. Arginine: The Nitric Oxide Source, 25

4. Ashwagandha: Laid-back Ayurvedic Lovemaking, 29

5. Catuaba: Coitus Catalyst, 33

6. Choline and CDP-choline: Pump up the Volume, 37

7. DHEA: Libido Life After Forty, 43

8. DMG and TMG: Triple Boost Your Lust, Today!, 49

9. Fish Oils: Lube Your Love Glands, 55

10. Ginseng: Renowned Asian Energizer, 61

11. Horny Goat Weed: Will it Make you Horny, too?, 67

12. Maca: Erotic Incan Herb From the High Andes, 71

13. Muira Puama: Brazilian Jungle Passion, 75

14. NADH: The Dopamine Connection, 79

15. Pregnenolone: Hormone of High Sensation, 83

16. Tongkat Ali: Exotic Asian Aphrodisiac, 87

17. Tribulus: Roadside Sex Weed that Works, 91

18. Yohimbe: Experience the Orgiastic Mating Rituals of the African Bantu, 97

19. Additional Sex Boosters: Potential Libido Lifts, 103

    Conclusion: Choosing the Sex Booster For You, 111

    References, 119

    Index, 131

Introduction

Understanding the Human Sexual Response

The act of making love can be one of the most important experiences of our lives. It offers intimacy, sensuality, pleasure, and gratification. It is also the means by which we create life. Unfortunately, for literally millions of men and women, sex is disappointing. If either you or your partner is one of those individuals who find sex more frustrating than fun—and you are looking for a more natural way to solve the problem—you've got the right book in your hands.

Natural Sex Boosters not only discusses aphrodisiac supplements for a lagging sex life, but also discusses supplements that can significantly enhance a normal sex life—for both men and women. It is possible to experience heights of sexual passion and enjoyment like you have never experienced or could imagine!

I personally prefer natural sex boosters to Viagra and other pharmaceutical medicines. Natural supplements such as the ones I will discuss help many aspects of the human sexual response, and have fewer side effects than prescription drugs.

NATURAL SEX BOOSTERS—HYPE OR REALITY?

Since time immemorial, people have been in search of foods, herbs, and potions meant to stimulate sexual desire and enhance lovemaking. The Egyptians, Greeks, Romans, Chinese, and others all had their favorite aphrodisiacs and herbal concoctions. We can thank Aphrodite, the Greek goddess of love, for the word "aphro-disiac." This preoccupation with finding love potions has existed throughout the centuries and up to the present time.

Shakespeare, in *A Midsummer Night's Dream*, writes:

Fetch me that flower, the herb I show'd thee once;
The juice of it on sleeping eyelids laid
Will make man or woman madly dote
Upon the next live creature that it sees.

The range of substances and methods recommended by sages of ancient cultures is mind-boggling. From ram's testicles to ground rhino horn, the pursuit of natural sex boosters has been an age-old quest with all the superstition and pseudo-science you might imagine, leading most scientists to dismiss such sexual enhancements as folklore. There is a general suspicion in the modern Western mindset that natural compounds purported to enhance sexual passion or performance are barely, if at all, effective. Most Westerners would be surprised to find out, however, that there are dozens of natural substances that enhance sexuality in both men and women—and some of them are quite powerful!

As medical science has given us a greater understanding of the human sexual response, research is beginning to uncover the biochemical mechanisms of how natural sex boosters actually work. I have searched through decades of published studies to bring to you a summary of these interesting research findings.

WOMEN AND SEX

Female sexual dysfunction is a common medical condition that can have a major impact on self-esteem, quality of life, mood, and relationships. While there are religious, sociological, and emotional elements to female sexual function and response, impairment can also occur due to medical problems. Female sexual dysfunction is often categorized into three major areas: lack of desire; problems with lubrication and sensation; and difficulty having an orgasm.

Declining sexual desire often troubles women as they get older, and is partly due to the body's decreasing levels of testosterone and other hormones. Testosterone powers the sex drive in both men and women. Stress or depression can also lead to low libido. Vaginal dryness can develop when estrogen levels drop as menopause approaches.

Many of the natural sex boosters discussed in this book work extremely well in women to enhance libido, arousal, lubrication, and sensation.

MEN AND SEX

In men, sexual dysfunction primarily takes the form of a decline in libido, and impotence. The 1992 National Institutes of Health (NIH) Conference on Impotence suggested "erectile dysfunction" (ED) as a more appropriate term for the inability to obtain and/or maintain penile erection sufficient for satisfactory sexual performance. ED is sometimes made worse by personal relationship issues. Male sexual dysfunction should be viewed as a chronic disease with medical, psychological, sociological, and behavioral components.

Common medical causes of ED include chronic illness or the side effects of drugs. Additional risk factors for ED include cardiovascular disease, smoking, obesity, and high cholesterol. Less commonly, the problem is psychological. Physical causes are more common in older individuals whereas psychological causes are more common in the young. Erectile dysfunction does not have to be a part of getting older. It's true that as you get older, you may need more stimulation (such as stroking and touching) to achieve an erection. You might also need to wait more time between erections. But older men need not accept sexual dysfunction as a normal consequence of aging.

MEDICAL EVALUATION OF SEXUAL DYSFUNCTION

Before embarking on any therapy for sexual dysfunction, it is a good idea to have a thorough medical evaluation and physical exam taken. Testing could uncover a physical cause of the sexual problem. A urinalysis, complete blood count and basic chemistry panel will help to rule out most metabolic diseases. In the elderly, because thyroid disease can manifest slowly, thyroid-stimulating hormone levels should be measured to rule out thyroid dysfunction. Additional tests recommended for those over the age of 55 with a history of low libido include blood levels of prolactin and testosterone. Excessive prolactin has a negative influence on libido.

THE MANY FACETS OF
THE HUMAN SEXUAL RESPONSE

The sexual response involves much more than merely the sexual organs. There are several major areas of the human body that play a part in sexual arousal. These include hormonal, vascular, neural, psychological, and chemical processes. Let's discuss each of these areas in detail.

Hormonal

Androgens, such as testosterone, are a major component of libido in men and women. Testosterone levels decline about one percent each year in men, which may contribute to lower sex drive with aging. Testosterone also declines with age in women. Women who have had surgical removal of the ovaries often notice a drop in sexual interest. Replacement of androgens can be helpful in those with age-related sexual dysfunction.

Most hormonal problems revolve around dysfunction of the hypothalamic-pituitary-gonadal axis and are associated with either excess prolactin or decreased testosterone levels. Prolactin, a hormone made by the pituitary gland, inhibits sexual response when produced in high amounts. Other hormonal disorders that may cause sexual dysfunction include hypothyroidism, hyperthyroidism, adrenal insufficiency, or the presence of excessive levels of adrenal corticosteroids.

Testosterone is available by prescription only. Over-the-counter hormones, such as DHEA and androstenedione, convert into testosterone and thus have a positive influence on sex drive. Pregnenolone is another over-the-counter hormone that may increase testosterone levels.

4

Vascular

Disruptions in the flow of blood to and from the penis are thought to be a common cause of male erectile dysfunction. For instance, medical conditions such as atherosclerosis (hardening of the arteries), high cholesterol, hypertension, or diabetes reduce blood flow to the penis and genital organs thus leading to difficulty with erection or genital swelling. Additional factors that can impede blood flow include penile injury, surgery in the pelvic or abdominal area, and sitting on a bicycle too long. Men who log several thousand miles a year on their mountain bikes suffer scrotal damage that could reduce their fertility. Vascular disruptions may also reduce blood flow to the female genital organs.

Neural

Nerve damage from disorders such as diabetes, multiple sclerosis, Parkinson's disease, and stroke affects the brain's ability to respond to sexual stimulation. In women, abdominal or pelvic operations can occasionally lead to nerve damage. Sexual dysfunction is common in men undergoing surgical treatment for prostate enlargement or cancer.

Psychological

The causes of psychological sexual dysfunction are so numerous that it is difficult to list them all. However, most often these causes are related to depression, performance anxiety, marital stress or relationship problems, life crisis, financial difficulties, religious repression, or some type of mental illness.

Psychological erectile dysfunction is suspected when a person is able to have spontaneous erections during sleep, but has difficulty doing so with a partner. Most erections at night occur during REM (rapid eye movement) sleep.

Depression often coexists with sexual dysfunction, and the medical treatment of depression with certain drugs can further worsen sexual symptoms or cause sexual problems in a person who did not experience them prior to treatment.

Chemical

A normal sexual response in men and women often begins in the presence of sexually oriented stimulation. When the mood and setting are right, the body responds by releasing a cascade of chemicals that direct the flow of blood into the sexual organs. In men, this rush of blood is directed into a pair of pockets, known as the corpus cavernosa, that run along the shaft of the penis and allow the penis to engorge and stiffen. In women, this blood flow leads to engorgement and lubrication of the organs as the body prepares for sexual intercourse.

Some of the well-known chemicals involved in enhancing the human sexual response are nitric oxide (NO), dopamine, and acetylcholine. Serotonin has an inhibitory effect on sexual interest.

Engorgement of the sexual organs is triggered by a unique neurotransmitter called nitric oxide (NO). NO is considered the most important factor for relaxation of penile blood vessels and corpus cavernosa. Normally, the blood flow to the penis is restricted due to contraction of the blood vessels. However, through the relaxation of these vessels, the flow of blood increases and leads to erections. Some natural sex boosters work by influencing either the production of NO, or by influencing the production of other chemicals that are involved in the sexual response. Smoking reduces blood flow to the genitals and reduces the formation of nitric oxide.

The chemistry of sex is important to understand in order to maximize the potential of natural supplements. I will discuss this issue further in the next chapter.

SEX-BUSTING DRUGS

Up to one quarter of cases of sexual dysfunction may be due to medicines prescribed for a medical or psychiatric condition.

Common pharmacologic causes include diuretics, anti-hypertensives, beta-blockers, sedatives and sleeping pills, anti-seizure medicines, anti-HIV drugs, antipsychotics and antidepressants. Over-the-counter medications such as antihistamines and decongestants also interfere with optimum sexual performance. Sedatives and sleeping pills reduce sensation of genital organs. Alcohol has a negative effect on the sex drive, and this effect increases with age.

Antidepressants of the SSRI (selective serotonin reuptake inhibitors) class are well known to cause sexual problems. SSRIs include Prozac, Zoloft, Paxil, and others. SSRI-induced sexual dysfunction affects up to 60% or more of individuals who take these drugs. Biochemical mechanisms that are likely to cause this sexual dysfunction include increased serotonin; decreased dopamine; blockade of cholinergic receptors; and inhibition of nitric oxide synthetase. In response to this side effect, some doctors suggest a wait-and-see approach, while others may decrease the dosage or recommend drug holidays. More aggressive strategies for treating SSRI-induced sexual dysfunction include changing antidepressants and adding certain sex boosters. Bupropion and mirtazapine are antidepressants that are less likely to cause sexual dysfunction.

The hair-growing drug finasteride (Propecia), which is also prescribed as Proscar for use in benign prostate enlargement, may at times reduce sex drive. Finasteride blocks the conversion of testosterone to its more active form dihydrotestosterone (DHT). And since DHT is more potent than testosterone, it is possible that finasteride users may experience a drop in sexual interest.

ABOUT VIAGRA

A number of therapies have been developed over the years to address impaired sexual response, including the injection of drugs into penile tissue to induce an artificial erection, vacuum constriction devices, penile implantation surgery, hormones, and drugs.

Sildenafil, better known as Viagra, approved by the FDA in 1998, has been the most popular medicine for the treatment of erectile dysfunction. Two other drugs, Levitra and Cialis, were introduced to the U.S. market in 2003. Levitra is purported to work faster than Viagra, and Cialis is being promoted as helping erections last longer. Viagra works very well in dilating blood vessels in the genital region, which leads to an erection or increased blood flow to the vaginal tissues. However, it does little to directly increase libido or sexual arousal. The effect of Viagra is often noticed within an hour after taking a pill of 50 mg or 100 mg, and ease of erection may last up to twelve hours. Side effects of Viagra include headache, flushes, nasal congestion or runny nose, malaise, nausea, changes in blood pressure, irregular heartbeat, visual disturbances including rare cases of blindness, and chest pain.

I personally find natural sex boosters quite effective and preferable to pharmaceutical drugs. They may not be as effective as Viagra and the other new drugs in inducing erections, but they enhance overall sensation, sex drive, and sexual enjoyment. Hence, the entire sexual experience is much more pleasant.

MY EXPERIENCE

As part of my research in writing this book, I did a thorough search on Medline, the database for all medical studies published in Western medical journals. I also searched on the internet and visited many health food stores to find ingredients and products promoted by vitamin companies as sex boosters.

After more than two decades of medical practice and reading medical journals, I have come to realize that results of studies do not often reveal the whole picture. Often, I have learned a great deal about the effects of a particular nutrient or herb by taking it myself. For instance, I discovered in 1995 that melatonin, the pineal hormone used for sleep, causes vivid dreaming. I had not come across any mention of this in scientific journals. I also discovered in 1998 that high doses of fish oil capsules enhance visual perception. This, also, had not been mentioned in the medical literature.

Research on some of the nutrients and herbs discussed in this book is quite limited. Hence, I thought you, the reader, would appreciate any type of anecdotal information. Much of the information in *Natural Sex Boosters* is unique since I mention my own personal experiences, along with feedback from my patients and friends who have tried these aphrodisiacs. I have taken almost all of these herbs, nutrients, amino acids, or hormones for varying periods of time and in various doses—and some in combinations. Taking these sex boosters for the purposes of writing a book was quite an enjoyable experience!

Please be aware that my response may be quite different from yours. You may or may not experience the same findings. There is a significant difference among humans on how they respond to different herbs, supplements, and drugs. Also, there are variations between products from different sources and companies.

Many studies have found that there is a high placebo effect when testing with sex boosters. This placebo effect can be as high as 25% or more, and makes the interpretation of studies involving natural aphrodisiacs or anecdotal reports from individuals quite challenging.

THE RIGHT DOSAGE?

Throughout the book, I will mention a range of dosages for each supplement. It is impossible to give exact dosage suggestions that would apply to everyone, since each person has a unique biochemistry. There are many factors that influence a response to a particular supplement. These include age, sex, race, mindset, setting, medical or psychological condition, other medicines or supplements that are taken at the same time, quality of the supplement, etc. Another factor to consider is that the amount of the active ingredients in an herb may vary according to the region in which it is grown, the type of soil, the method of harvesting, storage, the quality of the product itself, weather conditions, and a number of other elements. Furthermore, many of these botanicals have only just begun to be investigated for their sex-boosting effect and hence little is known about the proper dosage and timing.

As a rule, and to be on the safe side, start at the low end of the dosage suggestions and gradually build up depending on the way the substance makes you feel. Another basic rule is that most women will require a dose smaller than those recommended for men. Perhaps only one-half or two-thirds of the dosage for males will be needed for women.

A WORD OF CAUTION

It is very difficult to predict how you will respond to the sex boosters discussed in this book. If you have a concern due to a medical condition or are currently taking medication, discuss the issue with your health care provider before experimenting on your own. Please keep in mind that some of these natural sex boosters are quite powerful—particularly the hormones and yohimbe—and if misused they can cause unpleasant side effects. Concurrent use of supplements may mimic, magnify, or oppose the effect of medicines you may be taking. Herbs, even if natural, can be toxic if taken in excess.

Another factor to consider is that these natural sex enhancers may make you hypersexual, possibly changing the quality as well as the quantity of your sexual behavior and interests. There can be unpredictable allergic reactions to supplements or fillers in the capsules that may involve the lungs, heart, skin, or other organs. However, these allergic reactions are rare.

Since these natural supplements have rarely been tested in pregnant women, it would be best for such women to only use them under strict medical supervision. It is always important to weigh the possible benefits from taking a substance versus the potential side effects that may occur to the developing fetus.

HOW TO USE **NATURAL SEX BOOSTERS**

As a result of my research, I have gathered information on various herbs and natural supplements that have sex-boosting qualities. I have designed the following chapters to serve as a reference guide to help you discover the right aphrodisiac for you.

Chapter 1 contains a brief discussion of the chemicals that are involved in the process of sexual arousal. You will likely return to this chapter to refresh your understanding of the chemistry of sex. In Chapters 2 through 18, I include an alphabetical listing of the natural herbs that are most commonly available and promoted as sexual enhancements. These individual chapters are organized to provide a concise overview of the most current information on each supplement. I begin with a brief explanation of the particular herb or nutrient. I then present the findings of any research studies that are available, and describe the way in which the product works. I then share with you my personal experiences in using the herb, as well as feedback from my patients who have tried the sex booster.

I also include the inevitable cautions and possible side effects from using each product, and the suggested dosages for the various forms that may be available. Unfortunately, many of these nutrients have not been well studied in the Western medical literature, and there are few extended human trials on which to report. As a result, long-term side effects are largely unknown. In addition, there is a lack of specific dosage recommendations for these natural products, unlike the product labels of pharmaceuticals.

The field of natural sex boosters is an evolving one. That is why I have included Chapter 19. This chapter details some sex-boosting herbs that have been reported to have aphrodisiac qualities. These products often appear among the ingredients list on other labels. However, these herbs are not presented in individual chapters, as there is either a lack of research evaluating these herbs, or the nutrients do not provide an immediate sexual effect. Hopefully, future studies will provide greater insight into these herbs and their wondrous possibilities to enrich and enhance your sex life.

Over the past several decades, science has slowly become aware of the potential of natural supplements and herbs in influencing the human sexual response. The research in this field is still in a quite early stage, and much is yet to be discovered about the potential benefits of these supplements and their proper dosages and combinations. I am very pleased to share with you my findings regarding dozens of natural sex boosters. But first, in the next chapter, let me explain in greater detail the chemicals that influence stamina, sensation, and sexuality.

1.

Sex Chemistry Made Simple

All stimuli that arouse us sexually, whether through touch, vision, hearing, taste, or smell, are processed in the brain through electrical and chemical messengers. The chemical messengers that help nerve cells communicate with each other are called *neurotransmitters*. Dozens of chemicals in the brain and body—amino acids, hormones, coenzymes, and peptides—act as neurotransmitters, influencing mood, alertness, and sexual arousal. A review of all of these neurotransmitters is not necessary for the purposes of this book. However, a brief explanation of some of the important neurotransmitters involved in sex will make it easier to understand how natural sex boosters work. This understanding will help you choose the right supplements for your particular sexual needs.

Use this chapter as a reference. You will probably find yourself returning to it when you encounter a sex booster that is particularly helpful. If your desire involves learning more about the aphrodisiac, try delving into the biochemistry of sex in more detail.

CHEMICALS INVOLVED IN SEXUAL AROUSAL

- **Nitric oxide (NO)** is the most important chemical responsible for engorgement of sexual organs and erections.

- **Acetylcholine** helps facilitate erections.

- **Dopamine** is primarily responsible for enhancing sex drive, mood, alertness, and movement.

- **Norepinephrine and epinephrine** influence alertness, arousal, and mood. These neurotransmitters increase libido, but may make it more difficult to have an erection.

- **Serotonin** usually has an inhibitory effect, that is, too much serotonin decreases sexual drive and interest.

Please keep in mind that these definitions are simplifications. Neurotransmitters have different effects in different parts of the brain and body.

HOW AN ERECTION HAPPENS

An erection is a complex event that occurs when blood rapidly flows into the penis and becomes trapped in its spongy chambers, called the corpora cavernosa. In addition to psychological and chemical components, an erection involves the neural, hormonal, and vascular systems.

When visual or auditory stimuli of a sexual nature stimulate the brain, nerve impulses flow down the spinal cord where they activate parasympathetic nerve fibers, which go to the penis or clitoris and release acetylcholine. Acetylcholine helps cavernous smooth muscles to relax and as a result more blood flows to the penis. Touching the penis also stimulates the parasympathetic nerves. Usually, both mechanisms are at work to cause erections, but as people age, they derive less stimulation from the higher centers and need to rely more on direct penile or clitoral stimulation. In the young, higher centers of the brain are easily stimulated by fantasizing or thinking about sex, which seem to cause an erection or vaginal lubrication nearly at will. Another aging-related change is an increase in the refractory period, that is, the time from ejaculation to the next erection. This interval may range from several minutes in a young man to several days in a 90-year-old.

When the penis is flaccid, the muscles of the corpora cavernosa are in a contracted state. This is maintained by the sympathetic nervous system using the chemical norepinephrine, which binds to alpha-1-adrenergic receptors. Yohimbine, a substance found in the African sex booster yohimbe, blocks these alpha-1-adrenergic receptors and prevents the contraction otherwise induced by norepinephrine. Erections now occur much easier since the corpora cavernosa are relaxed and blood can rapidly flow in. Nitric oxide is another chemical involved in erections.

NITRIC OXIDE: SAY YES TO NO

Nitric oxide (NO) is the most important chemical involved in the engorgement of genital organs leading to erections. Throughout this book, you will find herbs and nutrients that help in the formation of this chemical. For instance, the amino acid arginine can be metabolized into NO by an enzyme known as nitric oxide synthase. This conversion is done in endothelial cells, which are cells that line the inside of blood vessels. Ginseng, the popular herbal aphrodisiac, is also thought to increase NO levels.

NO functions by activating an enzyme called guanylate cyclase. Guanylate cyclase, in turn, helps form cyclic guanosine monophosphate (cGMP). The chemical cGMP becomes the secondary messenger that causes smooth muscle relaxation, resulting in venous engorgement and erections.

Under normal conditions, cGMP helps the muscles surrounding the arteries of the penis and the muscles of the corpus cavernosum to relax. This allows blood to easily flow into the penis. Any condition that interferes with the signaling of these messenger enzymes can quickly lead to the breakdown of the entire process and cause erectile dysfunction. Viagra works by blocking an enzyme that breaks down cGMP, hence more of this chemical is left to help dilate the genital arteries. Interestingly, having adequate levels of androgen hormones in the body makes it easier for the genital organs to respond to nitric oxide.

DOPAMINE

Dopamine is one of the most important neurotransmitters involved in the human sexual response. Dopamine has a significant effect on sexual desire. Plus, elevation of dopamine levels often leads to an improvement in mood and alertness.

A number of psychiatric disorders, particularly Parkinson's disease and mood disorders, are attributed to imbalances in dopamine levels. Dopamine is made from the amino acid tyrosine. Once produced, dopamine can, in turn, convert into the brain chemicals norepinephrine and epinephrine. Some of the natural supplements that increase dopamine levels include NADH and CDP-choline.

ACETYLCHOLINE

Acetylcholine was the very first neurotransmitter to be identified back in the early 1900s. It is made simply from choline, a natural substance found in lecithin, and a two-carbon molecule called acetyl. Acetylcholine plays numerous roles in the nervous system. In the brain, acetylcholine is involved in learning and memory whereas in the genital organs, acetylcholine is released by the parasympathetic nerves. Acetylcholine helps in the release of nitric oxide, which leads to the relaxation of smooth muscles and engorgement of the genital organs. Nutrients that elevate levels of acetylcholine include choline and CDP-choline.

NOREPINEPHRINE

In the flaccid state of the penis, frequent release of norepinephrine from sympathetic nerves contracts the arteries in the penis and also contracts the smooth muscles of the corpora cavernosum. Therefore, in the normal state, norepinephrine keeps the penis soft. A relative predominance of norepinephrine-induced contraction over nitric oxide-mediated relaxation may contribute to the problem of erectile dysfunction.

Two amino acids, phenylalanine and tyrosine, sold as supplements, are converted into dopamine. Dopamine, in turn, is converted into norepinephrine, and then epinephrine. The ingestion of these amino acids elevates dopamine and norepinephrine levels, and hence will lead to alertness and mood elevation and increased sexual interest. However, excess amounts of norepinephrine and epinephrine may make it difficult to have erections. In addition, high amounts raise blood pressure, increase heart rate, and cause anxiety, irritability, and insomnia.

Yohimbe, the natural sex booster from Africa, facilitates erections by blocking the inhibitory action of norepinephrine on the penis. I will discuss yohimbe in detail in Chapter 18.

SEROTONIN

Serotonin happens to be the most widely studied neurotransmitter since it helps regulate a vast range of psychological and biological functions. Serotonin (5-hydroxytryptamine or 5-HT) was first identified in 1948. The wide array of psychological functions regulated by serotonin involves mood, anxiety, libido, aggression, and thinking abilities. You may recall that other brain chemicals, such as dopamine and norepinephrine, also influence mood and arousal. However, serotonin generally has different effects. For instance, excess amounts of serotonin cause relaxation, sedation, and a decrease in sexual drive.

Prozac, a common antidepressant of the SSRI type, elevates serotonin levels in the brain. One of the common side effects of SSRIs is diminished sexual urge and sensation. There is a nutrient called 5-hydroxytryptophan (5-HTP) that is the immediate precursor to serotonin. When ingested as a supplement, 5-HTP converts in the brain into serotonin. The substance 5-HTP is often used to treat depression and anxiety. I have noticed that 5-HTP supplements decrease sexual interest.

ADDITIONAL SEX CHEMICALS

There are dozens of other chemicals—amino acids, peptides, and hormones—that influence the human sexual response. These include endorphins, growth hormone, vasoactive intestinal peptide, oxytocin, prostaglandins, and others. It is very likely that many of the supplements discussed in this book affect these chemicals, and further research will certainly identify these biochemical processes.

EXERCISE AND BODY IMAGE

Exercise can keep your heart healthy, your body slim, and your psyche sound, and it can act as an aphrodisiac too. Physical fitness may indirectly improve sexual desire and performance. When you feel better about your body image, you are more likely to feel sexy. Exercise can also help you sleep more soundly. Deep sleep does wonders to a lagging sex drive. Many patients report to me that yoga—a form of exercise and meditation that involves holding postures, stretching, and relaxed breathing—enhances their sexual interest. Yoga also helps the body become limber and brings about a sense of calm. Personally, I have found that regular yoga practice enhances my libido.

NUTRITION AND SEX

Good nutrition often helps sexual dysfunction over time, either by revitalizing overall health and libido, or by improving blood flow to the genital organs. Contrary to popular belief, there is no scientific proof that specific foods, such as oysters, caviar, or champagne have an immediate effect on libido. However, it is possible that certain classes of foods—for instance cold-water fish such as salmon—due to their content of fish oils, may boost sexual health over time. The benefits of fish oils are discussed in greater detail in Chapter 9.

It is a good idea to eat a whole-foods diet that focuses on fresh vegetables and fruits, whole grains, fish, poultry, and flax seed, and to drink plenty of fresh water. Choose organically grown foods when possible. Avoid or reduce your intake of processed foods, fast foods, junk foods, animal fats, hydrogenated oils and margarine, sugar and white flour products, alcohol, and caffeine.

Throughout the centuries, people did not know the reasons why a particular herb enhanced the libido—only that it worked. I find sexual chemistry fascinating, particularly since we are now beginning to understand how natural sex boosters work on a biochemical level. This knowledge will help us to more reliably choose our supplements and improve our sexual enjoyment and stamina.

2. Androstenedione

The Father of Testosterone

Androstenedione and its close cousins androstenediol, norandrostenedione, and others, are natural steroid hormones found in the body and also available over-the-counter. There are several other steroid hormones available without a prescription, including DHEA and pregnenolone.

Basically, pregnenolone is the grandmother of all the steroid hormones. Pregnenolone is able to convert into DHEA, which in turn converts into androstenedione, or "andro" for short. The body can then transform andro into testosterone and estrogen.

Steroid hormones are made mostly in the adrenal glands, testicles (in men), and ovaries (in women). However, they can also originate in other parts of the body such as the brain, where they are called neurosteroids. Andro and testosterone are known as androgens, while DHEA is known as a pro-androgen since it converts into androgens. Since andro is the precursor to testosterone, there has been speculation that andro has libido-boosting properties.

WHAT THE RESEARCH SAYS

I could not find any research regarding the role of andro on libido. However, there have been countless studies supporting the role of other androgens, such as testosterone, in increasing sex drive and overall sexual enjoyment.

Androgens are known to enhance sexual thoughts and fantasies

19

as well as enhance mood and well-being. Androgens facilitate the action of nitric oxide in causing genital swelling, and they also enhance the sensation of genital organs such as the clitoris and penis. It is possible that androgens also increase the sensation of the nipples.

HOW IT WORKS

Since andro transforms into testosterone, it follows that it should have sex-boosting properties similar to testosterone. Most studies show that andro raises blood levels of testosterone and estrogens. In addition, andro enters cells of various organs and tissues in the body and converts to testosterone and estrogens within the cells.

MY EXPERIENCE

I personally have not taken andro because my skin is very sensitive to androgens. I break out in acne within a few days after taking DHEA or even pregnenolone. However, I have definitely noticed libido-boosting effects from DHEA and pregnenolone. In Chapters 7 and 15, respectively, I discuss the effects from using the hormones DHEA and pregnenolone.

REPORTS FROM PATIENTS

Carol, a 39-year-old personal trainer, took 25 mg of andro two mornings in a row. "I think I now know what it feels like to be a man," she says. "I couldn't keep my hands off my boyfriend. He was surprised how aggressive I became in bed."

A 57-year-old male architect says, "Andro increases my libido, promotes a feeling of well-being and helps with mental alertness."

Both male and female patients frequently report to me that they notice a libido-boosting effect from this hormone. Others find that they can ejaculate easier. Occasionally someone will notice the effect within an hour, but more commonly the sexual enhancement is noticed the next day or third day of use. Therefore, if you expect to be sexually active over the weekend, you could take andro Thursday and Friday.

On the other hand, and I don't know how to explain it, I have had reports from individuals who have noticed a decrease in sex drive while taking andro daily for many weeks.

A 32-year-old male patient says, "I tried andro 100 mg a day for three weeks while weight training and noticed no positive effects, and if anything my libido appeared to go down."

CAUTIONS AND SIDE EFFECTS

If you plan to take andro, do so under medical supervision, and take it for a maximum of a few days per month.

Most of the short-term side effects are not serious and include acne, mood changes, and irritability. These side effects are minimal with low dosages, particularly if andro is only taken for two or three days. Acne results from the increased production of sebum—the semi-liquid, greasy secretion of the sebaceous glands in the skin. I am aware of several reports of aggressive behavior by individuals taking andro.

When andro is taken for prolonged periods, it can have additional side effects that include thinning of scalp hair, facial hair growth in women, and alterations in menstrual cycles. Blurred vision is another side effect that a few andro users have experienced. Thinning of scalp hair may occur due to the transformation of andro into testosterone, which then converts in the hair follicles into dihydrotestosterone (DHT). Hair follicles do not like too much DHT. There's actually a hair-growth medicine called finasteride that works by blocking the conversion of testosterone to DHT. Andro can also raise levels of estrogen, which could potentially lead to enlarged breasts and an increased risk of certain types of cancer if taken daily for many years. Prostate enlargement is a potential concern in older men. I am aware that DHEA, in doses greater than 25 mg, sometimes causes irregular heart rhythms. It is possible that andro may do the same in susceptible individuals.

A letter to the editor of *The New England Journal of Medicine* reports an individual's experience as a result of taking andro for the purpose of improving his physique. He experienced priapism (painful continuous erection) for over thirty hours after taking the hormone for one week. The priapism required a visit to the emergency room. (Priapism is named after Priapus, the Greek god of fertility often shown in sculpture endowed with a large phallus.)

DOSAGE AND AVAILABILITY

Andro is available in health food and vitamin stores in 25, 50, and 100 mg capsules, but it is also available in other forms including percutaneous gels, transdermal patches, and chewing gum. Andro is often found in combination with other hormones, such as DHEA, and herbs such as tribulus. It is important to remember that combining andro with DHEA will have an additive effect. Taking andro with tribulus appears to be safe. A dose of 10 to 50 mg a day for one to four days is usually effective for most people as a sex booster. Those planning to start off by taking 10 mg would have to open a higher-dosage capsule to get the reduced amount. If taken in gel or transdermal patch form, be sure to follow the directions on the packaging label, as the concentration of andro will vary between different products. Some people find that taking a pill a couple of hours before sex is effective.

The young and those with high levels of androgens in their system are not likely to notice as much of a sex-boosting effect from andro as would middle-aged and older individuals. As with any supplement, some people will notice benefits while others may only experience side effects. It is difficult to predict a person's response to a nutrient, herb, or hormone. Andro seems to be most appropriate for those who have a low libido or who notice a decrease in genital sensation.

Androstenedione can be safely used in low dosages for short periods of time in order to enhance libido, particularly if taken under medical supervision. The dosage may vary between 10 mg and 50 mg per day for one to four days, followed by a break for several weeks. Those who are deficient in androgens due to a medical condition or aging could take andro or DHEA for prolonged periods—as long as they are monitored by a physician.

Taking andro for prolonged periods of time could potentially lead to serious side effects. Andro, being the immediate precursor to testosterone, is a controversial supplement in the eyes of the FDA, since it is available over-the-counter, while testosterone is a prescription medicine. The FDA frequently reviews safety data regarding this supplement to decide whether to keep it available to the consumer without a prescription.

The sex-boosting effects of andro and DHEA are somewhat similar and either can be used interchangeably. If you plan to use andro, note that other steroid hormones such as DHEA, pregnenolone, and others related to androstenedione, will have an additive effect if taken at the same time.

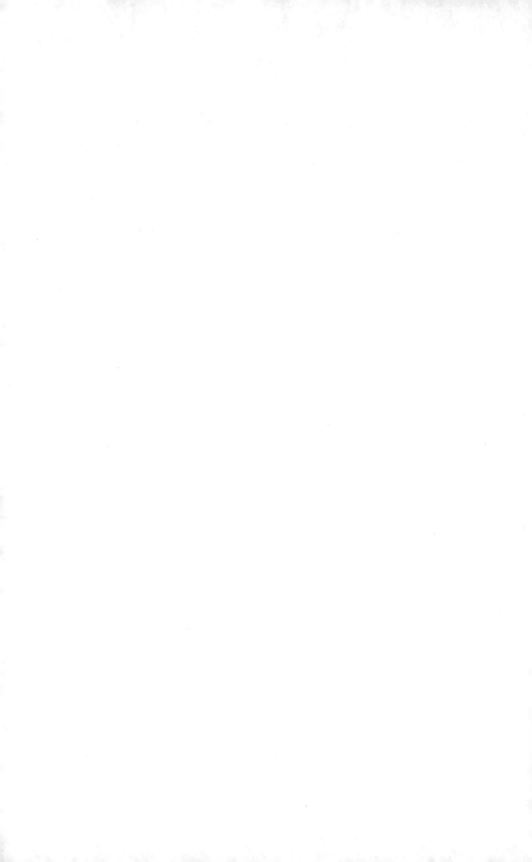

3. Arginine

The Nitric Oxide Source

One of the more highly advertised and promoted supplements used for the treatment of sexual dysfunction is L-arginine, also referred to as arginine. Arginine is a versatile amino acid in animal cells, serving as a precursor for the making not only of proteins but also of nitric oxide, urea, glutamate, and creatine. What makes arginine interesting is that it can be metabolized into nitric oxide (NO). Nitric oxide is the most powerful chemical known to dilate and engorge blood vessels of the penis and clitoris.

WHAT THE RESEARCH SAYS

Low doses of arginine, at 500 mg three times a day, have not been found to be effective. A double-blind, placebo-controlled study of fifty men with erectile dysfunction tested arginine at a dose of 5 g per day for six weeks. About one-third of the participants who received arginine showed improvement, but that improvement was greater than the 10% improvement seen in the placebo group.

Arginine has been studied in combination with other nutrients as a treatment for sexual dysfunction in women. A small trial found some improvement with a combination treatment (Argin-Max for Women) providing a daily dose of 2,500 mg of arginine, as well as ginseng, ginkgo, and damiana. In a four-week, double-blind study, seventy-seven women with decreased libido were given either the combination product or a placebo. Those taking the arginine-blend showed statistically greater improvement, reporting increased sexual desire in 71% of participants given the treatment. In the placebo group, 42% reported an increased libido. Other improvements included relative satisfaction with sex life and heightened clitoral sensation. No significant side effects were seen in either group.

A study done at the University of Texas at Austin examined the effects of arginine, combined with yohimbine, on sexual arousal in postmenopausal women. Twenty-four women participated in three sessions in which sexual responses to erotic stimuli were measured following treatment with either arginine glutamate (6 g) plus yohimbine (6 mg), yohimbine alone (6 mg), or a placebo, using a randomized, double-blind design. Sexual responses were measured at one hour after taking the supplements. Compared to the placebo, the combined oral administration of arginine and yohimbine substantially increased vaginal pulse amplitude responses to the erotic film.

Interestingly, a similar study using the same combination was tested at the Hopital Foch, Suresnes, in France. But this time, the study was done with forty-five men who had erectile dysfunction (ED). For a two-week period, the supplements were administered orally, two hours before intended sexual intercourse. Reports from this initial trial showed that the oral administration of the arginine and yohimbine combination is effective in improving ED.

In 2003, researchers in Bulgaria conducted a study in which subjects received a combination of arginine and pycnogenol. Pycnogenol is the product name of an extract made from the bark of the French Maritime Pine, which grows in Europe. It is a blend of bioflavonoids including catechin, epicatechin, taxifolin, oligomeric proanthocyanidnins, and phenolic fruit acids such as ferulic acid and caffeic acid. Many fruits and berries contain similar bioflavonoids. During the study, which lasted a period of three months, subjects received 1.7 g of arginine and 120 mg of pycnogenol each day. Researchers found this combination of arginine and pycnogenol to be helpful in young men, aged 25 to 40, who had psychological, but not organic, erectile dysfunction. However, it is difficult to say whether arginine was a significant factor in producing benefits or whether pycnogenol by itself would have been just as helpful.

HOW IT WORKS

The most likely explanation for the modest effectiveness of arginine is its conversion into nitric oxide. As discussed in Chapter 1, nitric oxide is converted into cGMP, which becomes the secondary messenger that causes smooth muscle relaxation, resulting in more blood going into the genital organs, which leads to erections. However, nitric oxide is metabolized quite rapidly, which may explain why taking arginine does not lead to consistent or prolonged erections.

MY EXPERIENCE

Low doses of arginine, such as less than 3 g, do nothing for me. I find than I need at least 6 to 10 g to notice an improvement in engorgement, but this effect is often short-lived. I have taken up to 14 g of arginine in one day with no apparent ill effects.

REPORTS FROM PATIENTS

The majority of people who take arginine by itself find that they need very high doses, such as a minimum of 6 g, to notice any benefits. In general, women do not seem to find arginine helpful enough to use.

Gary, a 50-year-old engineer, says, "I have read a lot about arginine for erectile dysfunction and I expected it to work really well, but I find that I need to take at least 10 g to notice an effect. This effect only lasts several minutes, unless I take it along with yohimbe. The combination works better for me."

CAUTIONS AND SIDE EFFECTS

The most common side effect noted is a mild feeling of flushing that comes on within the first hour of intake.

DOSAGE AND AVAILABILITY

Arginine is an amino acid available over-the-counter, usually in capsules ranging from 500 to 1000 mg, and also as a powder. If you plan to take arginine frequently, the powder is likely to be cheaper and more convenient. Arginine is best taken on an empty stomach with a small amount of water or juice. Since we cannot predict how a person will react to a particular supplement, it would be preferable for your first dose to be a maximum of 2 g. If you can tolerate two grams, then you may gradually increase it to five grams. Consult your health care provider if you plan to take higher doses. The effects, although mild, are noticed in about an hour or two following usage.

Arginine appears to offer only a slight benefit for sexual dysfunction in women, and in men with erectile dysfunction. The required dosages are quite high, usually ranging from a minimum of 5 to 10 g. Arginine by itself is a weak sex booster, and if used at all, it is better suited in combination with other herbs and nutrients. We can make full use of arginine's potential by combining it with other sex boosters. One option that has been supported by research is combining arginine with yohimbe, as discussed above. Arginine may also be combined with pycnogenol or other supplements that contain bioflavonoids.

4. Ashwagandha
Laid-back Ayurvedic Lovemaking

Ashwagandha is a shrub cultivated in India and North America whose roots have been used for thousands of years by Ayurvedic practitioners. In Ayurveda, the traditional Indian system of medicine, ashwagandha is used to promote physical and mental health, to provide defense against disease, and as a sexual tonic. Ashwagandha is sometimes referred to as Indian ginseng.

WHAT THE RESEARCH SAYS

Studies over the past few years indicate that ashwagandha has several interesting benefits. These include such positive effects as antioxidant, mind-boosting, anti-inflammatory, anti-tumor, anti-stress, and immune-enhancing properties.

Researchers from Banaras Hindu University in Varanasi, India, have discovered that some of the chemicals in ashwagandha are effective antioxidants. They tested these compounds for their effects on rats' brains and found an increase in the levels of three natural antioxidants—superoxide dismutase, catalase, and glutathione peroxidase. A human trial conducted at the same university found ashwagandha to be an effective mood stabilizer in those with anxiety and depression.

Additional studies indicate ashwagandha stimulates the growth of axons and dendrites, the parts of nerve cells that reach out from the nerve body to touch, connect, and communicate with other nerve cells. As of yet, no studies have been published directly evaluating the role of ashwagandha as an aphrodisiac.

HOW IT WORKS

Ashwagandha contains flavonoids and many active ingredients of the withanolide class, in addition to coumarins, triterpenes, and phytosterols. Little is known as to the possible mode of action of ashwagandha as a sex booster. One study shows that ashwagandha stimulates an enzyme known as nitric oxide synthase. This enzyme helps form nitric oxide, one of the important chemicals involved in dilating blood vessels to the genital organs. There are probably additional, yet undetermined, ways in which ashwagandha works as a sex stimulant.

Ashwagandha is used in India to treat mental deficiencies in geriatric patients, including amnesia. Researchers from the University of Leipzig in Germany wanted to find out which neurotransmitters were influenced by ashwagandha. After injecting some of the chemicals found in ashwagandha into rats, the researchers later examined slices of their brain and found an increase in acetylcholine receptor activity. As I mentioned in Chapter 1, acetylcholine is also involved in the process of dilation of blood vessels in the genital region.

As to its other properties, a study done at the University of Texas Health Science Center indicates that extracts of ashwagandha have GABA-like activity. GABA is a brain chemical involved in relaxation. This may account for this herb's anti-anxiety effects. Ashwagandha's botanical name, *Withania somniferum*, speaks of its sedative quality; *somniferum* means "sleep creator" in Latin.

It seems that the aphrodisiac properties of ashwagandha result from the stimulation of nitric oxide synthesis, and its effect on acetylcholine receptors. There are probably quite a number of additional undiscovered ways in which ashwagandha influences human biochemistry.

MY EXPERIENCE

I have taken several different ashwagandha products and noticed slight differences between them. Some produced a more sedating effect, while others caused alertness. These differences may be due to the age of the plant; the season in which it is picked; the type of soil; storage time; and also the extraction process—whether through water, alcohol immersion, or other means.

During one trial, I took a 500 mg ashwagandha pill at breakfast and lunch for one week. I felt calm and relaxed, and also noticed a mild increase in sexual interest. On another occasion, I took a one-time large dose of 3 g of ashwagandha, and noticed within several hours a more immediate effect, which involved easier erections.

REPORTS FROM PATIENTS

"Ashwagandha makes me feel like I want to continue touching myself," says Brad, a 42-year-old psychologist. "I take 500 mg twice a day."

Mary, 34, finds ashwagandha helps her in combination with other herbs. "When I combine ashwagandha with ginseng or yohimbe, the combination is much more effective. I get in the mood right away."

CAUTIONS AND SIDE EFFECTS

No significant side effects have been reported in the Western medical literature, but that does not mean that this herb is free of side effects. We just do not know enough about its long-term influence on the human body. Since some ashwagandha products have mild sedating properties, caution is advised if operating heavy machinery or driving long distances, particularly at night.

DOSAGE AND AVAILABILITY

A variety of dosages and forms of ashwagandha are available. Most commonly, extracts of the root are sold in capsules ranging from 200 to 500 mg, while the root is sold in capsules ranging from 500 to 1000 mg. Since the extract is more concentrated, less is required to achieve the desired effect. However, since different herb suppliers and product manufacturers provide various extracts and concentrates, it is difficult to give precise dosages.

Sometimes, the bottle will list that the product is standardized to a certain percentage of withanolides, most commonly 1.5%, although I have come across an extract of 5%. Withanolides are considered some of the active chemicals within ashwagandha. Whether the products with a higher percentage of extract offer additional benefits is not clear at this time. As to the overall health benefits regarding the regular ashwagandha powder versus the extract, no studies are available to provide any clues. In addition to capsules, this herb is available as a liquid extract.

An average daily dose is usually 1 to 3 g of the root, or 0.5 to 1.5 g of the extract. To prepare a tea, boil 3 to 6 g of the roots for fifteen minutes, and one to three cups may be drunk daily. Tinctures, or fluid extracts, can be used in the amount of 1 or 2 ml once in the evening, or three times a day for those who wish to enhance their sex life, in addition to having an herb that helps them with daytime anxiety.

If you are the type of person who is generally sluggish during the day, take ashwagandha towards the evening. If you happen to be over-energetic and hyper, you could take this herb anytime during the day. You could cycle the use of this herb by taking it two weeks on and then one week off. This is a rough guideline, however, as I generally suggest to my patients to take breaks from the use of a product just in case there are long-term side effects that we may not be aware of based on the limited scientific knowledge available.

Ashwagandha is an ideal aphrodisiac for those whose sexual dysfunction is partly due to anxiety. Most users will not notice a feeling of sedation, just a relaxed sense of laid-back Ayurvedic lovemaking. As an added bonus, ashwagandha can be combined with other sex boosters that have more of a stimulant nature, for example yohimbe, ginseng, choline, NADH, or DMG, all of which I will discuss in later chapters.

5. Catuaba

Coitus Catalyst

Catuaba (*Erythroxylum catuaba*) is a medium-sized tree found in the northern part of Brazil. In Brazilian herbal medicine, catuaba bark is considered a central nervous system stimulant with aphrodisiac properties. Historically, such a bark decoction has been used as a mind booster and sex booster, and for the treatment of fatigue.

WHAT THE RESEARCH SAYS

I found only one study on Medline regarding catuaba. Researchers in Japan found that catuaba extracts given to mice produced antibacterial and anti-HIV activity. There have been no human trials published in the North American medical literature.

HOW IT WORKS

The components found in catuaba include alkaloids (catuabine A, B, and C), tannins, aromatic oils and fatty resins, phytosterols, and cyclolignans. The way in which catuaba works is not yet known.

MY EXPERIENCE

I took 1 ml of catuaba tincture morning and midday for three days in a row. I noticed that my erections were easier to start and maintain, but I did not experience any other physical or mental effects.

REPORTS FROM PATIENTS

About one-half of patients to whom I have recommended catuaba reported a positive response, with an enhanced ability to maintain erections.

Dennis, 47, says, "I do find catuaba helps me have better erections after several days of use, and a friend told me to combine it with muira puama. The combination seems to be more effective. I had previously noticed that muira puama enhanced my libido, and since the catuaba helps with my erections, it seems logical to combine them."

CAUTIONS AND SIDE EFFECTS

There are no known side effects, however the use of catuaba in North America is relatively new. Little information is known about its long-term safety.

DOSAGE AND AVAILABILITY

Amazonian natives have historically consumed catuaba as a tea made from the bark. Indigenous Brazilians claim that after drinking one to three cups of tea steadily over a period of a few days or weeks, the first effects that occur are usually erotic dreams, and then an increase in sexual desire. Claims have been made that an alcohol tincture extract contains more of the active ingredients and provides better results, although I have not come across such research.

Capsules are sold consisting of a range from 500 to 1,000 mg. The recommended dose would be 1 to 2 g per day. One full dropper of the alcohol tincture can be taken twice a day with breakfast and lunch. Catuaba is commonly found in two-ounce liquid bottles; one milliliter provides about 500 mg.

Catuaba has been used traditionally in combination with muira puama. Personally, I have found that muira puama has a stronger effect on energy, mood, and overall sexual interest, and it seems logical to combine it with catuaba, which, to me, had a more direct effect on the genital region.

Catuaba can certainly be combined with many other herbs and nutrients, including tongkat ali, yohimbe, tribulus, and others. There are no specific guidelines for these combinations that would apply to everyone. It would be best to try catuaba, or any particular herb, on its own for a couple weeks until you understand how it works for you. Then, start taking lower doses of two herbs together to see how you respond to the combination.

6. Choline and CDP-Choline

Pump up the Volume

I came across the sex-boosting potential of CDP-choline by chance while writing my previous book *Mind Boosters*. I was very impressed by the effects of this nutrient.

Choline is a vitamin-like substance used as a precursor for making several important substances within the brain and body. Choline is widely available in a number of foods, particularly eggs, fish, legumes, nuts, and meats, as well as in human breast milk. Most individuals who have a normal diet are not deficient in choline, and dietary intake ranges from 300 to 900 mg a day. The importance of choline was emphasized in 1998 when the National Academy of Sciences classified it as an essential nutrient.

Choline has been sold over-the-counter for several decades. Choline is the forerunner to acetylcholine, one of the important chemicals involved in helping increase blood flow to the genital organs. Furthermore, the body can convert choline into TMG and DMG, libido boosters that I discuss in detail in Chapter 8.

A natural substance found within the body, CDP-choline (also called citicoline) had been available in Europe for a number of years before it became available over-the-counter in the U.S. in the late 1990s. In Europe and Japan, CDP-choline is approved for use in the treatment of stroke, Parkinson's disease, and certain other neurological disorders. CDP-choline, which stands for cytidine 5'-diphosphocholine, is an intermediary substance between choline and phosphatidylcholine (PC), also known as lecithin. In a simplistic way, you could consider CDP-choline a more potent and active form of choline.

There are many agents in clinical use that manipulate central nervous system levels of epinephrine, dopamine, and serotonin. However, development of pharmacological options to manipulate acetylcholine systems has lagged behind because of poor penetration of the blood-brain barrier and significant peripheral nervous system side effects. Fortunately, CDP-choline is one of the few agents that has the ability to influence brain levels of acetylcholine with fewer side effects than previous cholinergic medicines.

WHAT THE RESEARCH SAYS

I have not come across research directly evaluating the influence of choline or CDP-choline on libido or sexual performance. Most of the research with CDP-choline has been conducted in relation to its effectiveness in reducing brain damage following a stroke, and its potential use in the treatment of Alzheimer's disease. The research is still unclear as to whether CDP-choline plays a significant preservative role in stroke patients. However, newer research on retinal tissue cultures shows CDP-choline has a protective effect on damaged retinal nerve cells and has beneficial effects on the function of the brain visual pathway, mostly by enhancing the transmission of the neurotransmitter dopamine. Dopamine is an interesting brain chemical; higher levels lead to enhanced mood, better vision, and increased sex drive. A study in which 1,000 mg of CDP-choline was injected intramuscularly in patients with amblyopia for two weeks showed them to have improved visual acuity. Amblyopia is the term for loss of visual acuity in the non-dominant eye caused by lack of use of the eye in early childhood.

Phosphatidylcholine (PC) levels in brain cell membranes decrease with age. Evidence from both animal and in vitro studies indicates that CDP-choline administration increases the production of PC and other phospholipids in the brain, and might reverse the normal loss of PC with the aging process. Brain scans of older subjects, following being given 500 mg of CDP-choline for six weeks, were found to show a higher amount of PC and other phospholipids in the brain cell membranes. Nerve cells function better and communicate with each other in an enhanced way when the amount of phospholipids in their cell membranes is preserved. Therefore, the administration of CDP-choline could have some age-reversing effects on brain cells.

HOW THEY WORK

Choline can be converted into acetylcholine, a neurotransmitter that helps relax blood vessels involved in blood flow to the genital organs. See Chapter 1 for further details on the subject.

CDP-choline has many interesting biochemical activities that may explain why it has a sex-boosting effect. CDP-choline provides choline for the synthesis of the neurotransmitter acetylcholine. In addition, CDP-choline helps the release of the brain chemical dopamine, which is directly involved in increasing libido.

Over the years, many researchers have wondered whether CDP-choline, when ingested as a supplement, is absorbed intact and directly travels to the brain, or is first broken down and metabolized to other molecules before crossing into the brain. It is now thought that CDP-choline undergoes a quick transformation to cytidine and choline in rats, and uridine and choline in humans, which enter brain cells separately and possibly rejoin. It is difficult to say how this transformation influences sexual activity, since scientists are just now beginning to understand the way in which CDP-choline works.

MY EXPERIENCE

Within a few hours of taking choline, I experience enhanced mental focus, while erections become easier to maintain. I have not encountered side effects with amounts less than 500 mg. At dosages above 500 mg, I have noticed increased body warmth and sweating.

Within two hours of taking 500 mg of CDP-choline on an empty stomach, I find myself feeling more alert and motivated. In addition, colors seem brighter and sharper and I become more interested in sex, while erections last longer and are easier to maintain.

The sex-boosting effects are more apparent at 750 mg. Because of the alertness it produces, I have difficulty sleeping if I take this nutrient in the late afternoon or evening. Therefore, it would be best to take choline or CDP-choline no later than midday.

REPORTS FROM PATIENTS

Sylvia, 33, says, "I like choline since it is inexpensive and it works for me within four hours. One of the first things I notice is a slight increase in body warmth and then I realize my private parts seem more sensitive."

Greg, who is 40, has used CDP-choline off and on for several weeks. He reports, "I take 500 mg of CDP-choline three hours before sexual activity. My erections last longer and come easier. I also feel more alert."

CAUTIONS AND SIDE EFFECTS

A high intake of choline and CDP-choline is associated with mild gastrointestinal distress, nausea, sweating, increased body temperature, and loss of appetite. Toxicology studies show that CDP-choline produces no serious side effects in doses ranging from 500 mg to 1,000 mg a day when given for a few weeks. Long-term safety is not known, although one human study providing 1,000 mg of CDP-choline to patients with dementia for a one-year period did not indicate any significant side effects.

DOSAGE AND AVAILABILITY

Choline is sold in vitamin stores in doses ranging from 250 to 500 mg. It is available in a number of forms including choline bitartrate, choline chloride, and choline citrate. For practical purposes, choline may be taken in any of these forms. CDP-choline is commonly sold containing 250 mg per capsule. You may notice a sex-boosting effect within a few hours after taking 250 mg on an empty stomach, but taking higher amounts, such as 500 or 750 mg, is more consistently effective.

CDP-choline is a promising beneficial nutrient and I suspect that, with time, it will become more popular. Eventually science may find a role for it in the therapy of neurological conditions such as Alzheimer's disease, and perhaps Parkinson's disease. As to its aphrodisiac effect, it is a good supplement to have around for a quick sexual boost. CDP-choline is a good option for those who do not tolerate yohimbe, another fast-acting sex booster. I like the sex-boosting effects of choline also, but I find CDP-choline to be slightly more powerful. However, choline is much less expensive than CDP-choline.

7. DHEA

Libido Lift
After Forty

Dehydroepiandrosterone, or DHEA, is a hormone made mostly by the adrenal glands, but it is also produced in the testicles, ovaries, and the brain. Whether it is made by the body or ingested orally as a supplement, DHEA travels through the bloodstream and enters tissues and cells where it is converted to androstenedione, testosterone, and estrogens. The major circulating androgens in the blood include DHEA, androstenedione, testosterone, and dihydrotestosterone (DHT), in descending order of serum concentration. This means that the most prevalent androgen in the bloodstream is DHEA, and DHT is found in the least amount.

When we are young, our body produces appropriate amounts of hormones. However, the production of many hormones declines with aging. The production of pregnenolone, DHEA, growth hormone, progesterone, estrogen, and testosterone—all of which play an integral role in the sexual response—decreases with age.

Since DHEA converts into testosterone, and testosterone increases sex drive, I consider DHEA a powerful natural sex booster. In my clinical experience, at least one-half of the men and women who take DHEA report an increase in sex drive and sexual enjoyment, along with enhanced sensation. If used appropriately, DHEA can also lead to improvements in learning, memory, mood and energy, speed of thinking, concentration, awareness, and sensory perception.

The decline of hormone production can have a negative impact on a variety of bodily systems. Unfortunately, the field of hormone replacement is quite complicated and controversial, and there are no accepted medical guidelines at this time. For the purposes of this book, hormones are recommended only for occasional use as sex boosters, and not for life-long, continuous therapy.

WHAT THE RESEARCH SAYS

In 2002, Swedish researchers conducted a placebo-controlled, double-blind study. Researchers gave thirty-eight women, aged 25–65 years with androgen deficiency due to hypopituitarism, 30 mg of DHEA daily for six months. The ingestion of DHEA raised the blood levels of DHEA to normal age-related reference ranges and increased androstenedione and testosterone levels. The women on DHEA had improved alertness, stamina, and sexual interest. According to their partners, sexual relations tended to improve.

Dehydroepiandrosterone may be used occasionally by women who are sexually healthy. In a study conducted at the University of Washington in Seattle, sixteen sexually functional postmenopausal women participated in a randomized, double-blind trial in which they received 300 mg of DHEA or placebo sixty minutes before the presentation of an erotic video. Blood DHEA changes and subjective and physiological sexual responses were measured in response to videotaped neutral and erotic video segments. The concentration of DHEA increased two to five times following DHEA administration in all sixteen women. Subjective ratings showed significantly greater mental and physical sexual arousal to the erotic video with DHEA versus placebo.

Is DHEA as effective a sex booster in men as it is in women? A study conducted at the University Hospital Wurzburg in Germany showed that providing 50 mg of DHEA to men aged 50 to 69 years for four months did not lead to heightened sexual stimulation. However, a study completed at the Department of Urology within Austria's University Hospital of Vienna indicated that men with erectile dysfunction due to hypertension or unknown causes noticed improvement in sexual function when given 50 mg of DHEA for six months.

HOW IT WORKS

In contrast to the many herbs discussed in this book whose biochemical mechanism of action is not well understood, DHEA's influence on sex drive is quite clear. DHEA converts into such powerful androgens as androstenedione and testosterone. As previously discussed, testosterone is an important hormone mostly responsible for the libido in both men and women. Androgens also facilitate the action of nitrous oxide in the genital region, leading to easier genital engorgement and erections.

MY EXPERIENCE

I notice an enhancement in libido with DHEA, along with an improvement in skin sensation, which occur most often during my second or third day of use. My daily dose has been 10 mg. Unfortunately, even though I like the sex-boosting effect of DHEA, I break out in pimples and this limits my use.

REPORTS FROM PATIENTS

Judy, a 52-year-old travel agent married for twenty-four years, was having problems with her marriage. She told me, "A few years ago, I noticed a distance develop between me and my husband. I just didn't have the urge to be intimate; and obviously, this hurt our closeness. The problem was getting worse and I really thought we were going to break up. I started on 5 mg a day and within a week I couldn't keep my hands off my husband. He loved it. Now I only take the DHEA three or four times a month."

Many men also like the libido-enhancing benefits of taking DHEA. Michael, a 52-year-old lawyer, reported, "I've been having trouble getting excited lately. Maybe it's from the stress at work. I tried 25 mg of DHEA Thursday, Friday, and Saturday mornings. On Saturday evening, I got into bed with my wife. She gave me a little massage in the right places, and I could tell that my sensation was enhanced. I actually got more turned on than I had been for months!"

CAUTIONS AND SIDE EFFECTS

Dehydroepiandrosterone in low doses is safe, and side effects are minimal when used for only a few days. The side effects include acne, irritability, and aggressiveness. These unpleasant effects are clearly dose-dependent, and generally begin at doses above 10 mg. Individuals prone to acne, however, can get pimples from as low a dose as 2 mg. An infrequent side effect of high doses of DHEA, generally more than 15 mg, is heart palpitations—particularly in those prone to arrhythmias. A prescription medicine called propranolol, at a dose of 40 mg, is helpful in controlling or stopping the arrhythmia once it occurs.

Long-term use of DHEA could lead to menstrual irregularities, headaches, and mood changes. Women can experience facial hair growth. DHEA could potentially accelerate scalp hair thinning due to its conversion into DHT, the hormone associated with hair loss. If you experience hair loss, stop taking the DHEA and ask your doctor whether temporary therapy with finasteride, or Propecia, might be appropriate. Finasteride blocks the conversion of testosterone to DHT.

Those considering taking DHEA daily for many years should realize that there is a possibility that prolonged use may initiate or promote tumors, especially hormone-sensitive tumors. DHEA could also potentially increase the risk for a condition called benign prostate enlargement.

DOSAGE AND AVAILABILITY

DHEA is sold in pill or cream form, and is available as sublingual or timed-release pills. Pills are sold in dosages of 5 mg upwards to 100 mg. I hope more vitamin companies will begin to provide the 5 mg pills and stop selling products containing higher dosages. For the cream products, the label should list instructions and the amount of DHEA present per gram. It is possible that the sublingual tablets may be preferable since the DHEA would go directly into the bloodstream, as opposed to passing through the liver and intestines, where it would be partially metabolized. However, as there are no studies comparing the different products, it is difficult to make a firm recommendation as to what form of DHEA is the most effective.

Many individuals, especially those whose adrenal glands produce low levels of DHEA, notice an improvement in mood and sex drive when taking DHEA. Some report an improvement in stamina and concentration abilities. However, due to its potential side effects, the use of DHEA is best when limited to a few days per month. Medical supervision is recommended for people who wish to take hormones, even if these hormones are available over-the-counter. Due to age-related hormone decline, DHEA is most suitable for people of middle age and older.

8. DMG *and* TMG

Triple Boost Your Lust, Today!

U nless your major in college was chemistry, chances are you don't remember learning about methyl donors. But if you find the field of sex nutrients and mind-boosting pills interesting, you will certainly want to learn more about supplements that have the ability to be methyl donors. A methyl donor is simply any substance that can transfer a methyl group (a carbon atom attached to three hydrogen atoms, or CH3) to another substance. This transference, methylation, is a biochemical process that is essential to life, health, and regeneration of body cells. Vitamins, hormones, neurotransmitters, enzymes, nucleic acids (DNA and RNA), and antibodies depend on the transfer of methyl groups to complete their synthesis. It's quite likely that our body's ability to methylate declines with age.

Nutrients that have the capacity to be methyl donors include dimethylgycine (DMG), trimethylglycine (TMG), S-adenosyl-methionine (SAMe), and choline. Two of the B vitamins, folic acid and B12, are also considered to be methyl donors. Since methyl donors help the production of several neurotransmitters, they have an influence on sexual enjoyment, mood, energy, alertness, concentration, and visual clarity.

WHAT THE RESEARCH SAYS

DMG is found in very small amounts in some foods, such as cereal grains, beans, seeds, and liver. DMG has been available as a supplement since the 1970s, however its sex-boosting effect has not been studied.

Over the years, small-scale animal and human studies have indicated that DMG has immune system-boosting properties, enhances physical and mental performance, and has cardiovascular benefits. DMG also helps lower blood levels of homocysteine, a substance known to cause hardening of the arteries. Anecdotal reports indicate that DMG may be helpful in autism. Methyl donors have such a wide range of biochemical activities that many more studies are needed to confirm these results, and to determine their full clinical role in medicine.

Dietary sources of TMG include legumes, beets, and fish. Several studies show TMG, also known as betaine, helps lowers homocysteine levels, protects liver cells from toxins, and improves the health of those with a liver condition known as nonalcoholic steatohepatitis. The sex-boosting potential of TMG has not been formally studied.

HOW THEY WORK

DMG is basically the amino acid glycine attached to two methyl groups, while TMG has three methyl groups. Choline (tetramethylglycine) has four methyl groups, and when it donates a methyl group it becomes TMG. When TMG donates a methyl group it becomes DMG. DMG, in turn, has two methyl groups left to methylate other substances in the body.

DMG acts as a building block for the synthesis of many important substances such as choline, SAMe, the amino acid methionine, several hormones, neurotransmitters, and DNA. The formation of norepinephrine and dopamine requires a methyl group donated by SAMe. You may recall from Chapter 1 that dopamine enhances sex drive. Since DMG and TMG are methyl donors, which are instrumental in the production of various hormones and neurotransmitters, these two nutrients play an important role in sexual pleasure and mood.

MY EXPERIENCE

I definitely notice a sense of well-being, alertness, mental sharpness, and enhanced sexual interest and pleasure from both TMG and DMG, generally at a dose between 300 to 750 mg. The effects of sublingual DMG start within an hour.

I have tried DMG on several occasions, and each time the results have been consistent. Within an hour, I notice feeling more alert with a slightly sharper vision, and several hours later I experience a sense of well-being. The sex-boosting effects, which I usually notice within several hours or even a day or two of taking DMG, consist of having greater interest in sex, better erections, and stronger ejaculations.

After taking a rather high dose of DMG, I experienced mild nausea, which dissipated quickly. One morning, I consumed a large amount of TMG, which produced an energetic feeling that lasted through the night, up until the next day. The sexual effects from TMG usually take from a few hours to a day or two to notice, and are similar to DMG.

REPORTS FROM PATIENTS

Barbara, who is 52, had a quick response to sublingual DMG. "I felt more alert and noticed a slightly clearer vision within a half hour of melting 250 mg of DMG under my tongue," she says. "It was several hours later that I realized I was having more sexual thoughts."

Andy, 43, says, "I took 500 mg of TMG for three days in a row and I can attest that it had libido-boosting effects. I was thinking about sex more often than I normally do, and it seemed my genital organ sensation was enhanced."

CAUTIONS AND SIDE EFFECTS

TMG and DMG, if taken in high dosages, can cause nausea, elevated body temperature, sweating, restlessness, irritability, and general malaise. Insomnia may occur if DMG and TMG are taken in the evening. High doses of TMG, even when consumed in the morning, may cause insomnia. Low doses of these nutrients taken early in the day may actually provide a deeper sleep that night, since the alertness wears off by nighttime. The highest dose of DMG that I have taken is 1,000 mg. I experienced mild nausea and a feeling of unease, which lasted less than an hour.

One morning, I took three 750 mg pills of TMG (totaling 2,250 mg) on an empty stomach with an ounce of fruit juice just to see if there were any side effects. An hour later I felt the onset of nausea. Drinking a few ounces of milk relieved the nausea. As the day progressed, I felt more energetic and realized that my mood was enhanced. In the evening, I took my routine three-mile walk and noticed that I had a great deal of energy. I kept walking and ended up covering twice my normal distance. The drawback was that by bedtime I was still vitalized and couldn't sleep at all. I got out of bed several times throughout the night. I continued feeling the alertness well into the morning of the next day. Apparently, the very high dose of 2,250 mg can have effects on the brain that last more than twenty-four hours.

Your dose of TMG and DMG should be reduced if you are taking B vitamins, SAMe, DMAE, or choline, since these nutrients have overlapping functions. Since the nutrients TMG and DMG increase body temperature, avoid using them on particularly hot and humid days.

DOSAGE AND AVAILABILITY

DMG is available in many health food stores in small, foil-sealed 125 and 250 mg tablets. These tablets are melted in the mouth. Chewable tablets and liquid DMG are also sold. Capsules containing 100 mg have also been introduced. For a quick sex-boosting effect, take 500 mg sublingually. The suggested dosage of DMG for men is 250 to 500 mg, while women may benefit from only 100 to 250 mg. Since long-term studies on the use of DMG and TMG are not available, it would be best to take large doses of these supplements primarily only as needed for sexual enhancement. However, it appears that small doses, such as 100 mg or less, could be taken for more prolonged periods.

TMG is sold in tablets ranging from 250 to 750 mg. Men may

need to take 300 to 1,000 mg of TMG for one to three days to notice its full sex-enhancing effect. Women may notice the libido-boosting effects with a lower dose, such as 200 to 400 mg.

TMG and DMG are underutilized nutrients that hold a great deal of promise in health maintenance. Unfortunately, few doctors are familiar with these supplements. Since the body's ability to methylate declines with age, supplements of TMG or DMG in small amounts, such as 50 to 100 mg a day, may benefit middle-aged and older individuals.

I find DMG and TMG to be excellent natural sex boosters. For best results, you may need to take them for at least two or three days. A good option is to split your daily dose by taking half in the morning and the other half at noon. These nutrients should definitely be considered in any sex-boosting strategy.

9. Fish Oils

Lube Your Love Glands

Fish oils are found in such cold-water fish as salmon, halibut, and tuna. They have a beneficial effect on a number of medical conditions including heart disease, depression, stroke, autoimmune diseases, and dermatological disorders. Fish and fish oils have been promoted as brain foods. Are they potentially sex foods, too?

Fish oils contain omega-3 fatty acids called eicosapentanoic acid (EPA) and docosahexanoic acid (DHA). These fatty acids are an essential component of cell membranes in most organs and tissues of the body. They are also required for the normal development of the brain, the eyes, and the reproductive system. Interestingly, fish oils are found in semen. About sixty percent of the brain consists of lipids (fats), which make up the lining, or cell membrane, of every brain cell. The types of fats present in the brain influence its structure and function. How well your mind works depends, in the long run, on what you eat. A healthy brain is a prerequisite for a healthy sex drive.

WHAT THE RESEARCH SAYS

There is very little research available that provides an indication of the relationship between fish oils and sexual function. A thorough Medline search revealed only one study that gives us a hint. In this study conducted at Swallownest Court Hospital in Sheffield, England, the anti-depressive effect of ethyl-EPA was tested. Ethyl-EPA is the ethyl form of EPA, one of the two important fatty acids in fish oils. (Ethyl is a simple chemical comprised of two carbon atoms and five hydrogen atoms. It forms the base of common alcohol, ether, and other compounds.) Patients with persistent depression, despite ongoing treatment with an adequate dose of a standard antidepressant, were randomized on a double-blind basis. They were given either a placebo or 1 g ethyl-EPA per day for twelve weeks, in addition to their existing medication. No serious adverse effects were noted. Those taking ethyl-EPA were found to have an improvement in their depression, anxiety, and sleep pattern. Interestingly, they also reported having an improved libido!

Each capsule of fish oil normally sold over-the-counter has about 180 mg of EPA. Therefore, in the study above, the patients received an amount of EPA approximately equivalent to that found in about five capsules of fish oil.

HOW IT WORKS

It is unclear at this point exactly how fish oils influence sexuality. There may be several mechanisms involved. One possibility is that fish oils may help the formation of androgens in genital organs. A study with mice shows that a diet supplemented with fish oil influenced androgen formation in the testis differently than a diet with lard or coconut oil. Animals fed fish oils have healthier sperm.

Another possibility is that fish oils may improve circulation of the blood in the genital region. Several studies have shown that fish oils significantly improve the health of the cells lining blood vessels. They help these vessels dilate, produce more nitric oxide, and also produce more favorable prostaglandins. These protaglandins are hormone-like substances that help circulation in small blood vessels. Nitric oxide is the most important chemical involved in dilation of the blood vessels of genital organs, including the corpus cavernosa of the penis.

A third possibility is that fish oils may positively influence certain parts of the brain involved in the sexual response. The fact that the fatty acid DHA forms part of the cell membrane of brain cells indicates that the ingestion of fish oils could improve the health of brain cell membranes. This vitality could facilitate interaction and communication in the hypothalamus, pituitary, and other parts of the brain involved in maintaining proper hormone balance.

MY EXPERIENCE

I learned a great deal about the effects of fish oils while writing my previous book *Mind Boosters*. As an experiment, I took between five and ten capsules of fish oils per day for several days. I noticed within a couple of days that my vision had become sharper and clearer. After a few more days, I also realized that my interest in sex had increased and that I had more frequent spontaneous erections.

I have taken fish oil capsules on and off for several years, and each time I have noticed similar effects of improved vision within a couple of days, followed several days later by a heightened interest in sex. I have also noticed a slight enhancement in well-being and a mild sense of relaxation. It usually takes at least five capsules of fish oils per day for a minimum of three days for me to recognize these beneficial effects.

I have also experimented with very high daily dosages. The highest amount I have taken in one day is thirty capsules, each containing 300 mg of a combination EPA and DHA, totaling 9,000 mg. I took this dose in the morning, and by late afternoon I noticed the onset of clarity in vision, with objects looking sharper and clearer. There was a slight improvement in distance vision, and details became more noticeable. Fine print became easier to read. On the following day, I experienced the sex-boosting effects of consuming this high dosage. The visual improvement continued on subsequent days when I kept taking between ten to twenty capsules. Fish oil supplementation also makes me more serene, focused, and balanced. The effects, though, are subtle. I currently take about 600 to 900 mg of a combination EPA and DHA most days, except on days when I eat fish. This is equivalent to two or three capsules of fish oil.

REPORTS FROM PATIENTS

About one-third of my patients notice the positive effects of fish oils on libido.

One of my patients reports, "I have noticed an increased libido and have become more easily aroused since I've added fish and fish oils to my diet. I find that my erections come easier and I can maintain them longer. I think even the composition of my semen seems to have changed and has become thicker and creamier."

Gina, who is 29, is mostly vegetarian and does not like the taste of fish. She reports, "I believe it was the third day of taking eight fish oil capsules daily when I realized that more sexual thoughts were coming to me. I approached my husband in the kitchen—and he's the one who normally approaches me. When we started kissing, I felt much more aroused than usual."

CAUTIONS AND SIDE EFFECTS

The most common side effects from taking fish oils are mild indigestion and a fishy taste in the mouth. Fish oil supplements may interact with aspirin, non-steroidal anti-inflammatory drugs (NSAIDs) such as ibuprofen, and warfarin, or other anti-clotting medications, to cause excessive bleeding. Due to the fact that these oils can thin the blood, it is possible that very high doses could increase the risk of bleeding.

DOSAGE AND AVAILABILITY

Most fish oil capsules contain one gram of oil of which 120 mg is DHA, and another 180 mg is EPA. As a routine supplement, you could take one or two fish oil capsules a day for general health benefits, or perhaps three or four if you don't eat fish. For a sex-boosting effect, you may need to take five to eight capsules per day for a week. If you eat cold-water fish at least twice a week, you may not need to take fish oil capsules for health maintenance.

Fish oils can easily become rancid. Store the bottle in the refrigerator to slow the rate of oxidation. Opened bottles can be safely stored in the refrigerator for at least several weeks.

At this point, it is difficult to give precise dosages of fish oils that would apply to everyone. Individuals vary in their requirement for these fatty acids, depending on their dietary intake. As a rule, eating fish three times a week supplies about seven grams of EPA/DHA. A reasonable approach for someone who does not eat fish is to supplement with two or three fish oil capsules on a daily

What about Flaxseed Oil?

Flaxseed oil has a high percentage of a fatty acid called alpha-linolenic acid (ALA), which is able to convert into EPA. Since ALA in flaxseed oil can convert into EPA and DHA, why not just take flaxseed oil supplements instead of fish oils? This is a good option for those who are vegetarian and prefer flaxseed to fish oils. However, some people may not have the adequate biochemical ability to convert ALA into EPA. The conversion is a difficult process and may require more than 10 g of ALA to make 600 mg of EPA. The enzymes that convert less-saturated fatty acids such as ALA into EPA may not work efficiently in everyone. It has been suggested that several conditions or situations may cause inadequate activity of the enzymes that convert ALA into EPA and DHA. These conditions include aging, diabetes, intake of trans-fatty acids, and a large intake of saturated fatty acids.

My experience with flaxseed oil has been positive. When I take one tablespoon or more, I find that I have more energy and greater clarity of vision. This seems to improve over the following days if I continue taking the flaxseed oil. At higher doses, such as two tablespoons, I become overstimulated. I have not evaluated the influence of flaxseed oil on sexuality.

Based on the available evidence, it appears that most adults are able to convert ALA found in flaxseed oil to EPA, but some individuals are unable to do so adequately. Therefore, just to be on the safe side, it would seem reasonable to include flax oil in the diet, yet also to eat fish or take fish oil supplements. This way, all essential omega-3 fatty acids such as ALA, EPA, and DHA would be ingested.

basis. For faster sexual results, take five to eight fish oil capsules daily, and such benefits as increased libido and sexual enjoyment can be expected in a few days.

Individuals with a diet low in intake of seafood or foods supplying omega-3 fatty acids are likely to benefit from supplementation with fish oils or flaxseed oil. Unlike yohimbe, CDP-choline, or other sex boosters that provide a noticeable and pronounced effect within hours, the effects of fish oils are subtler and take longer to surface. If you are patient and can wait two or more days, then take the time to explore the benefits of fish oils. As with many of the herbs and nutrients discussed, it is a good idea to take breaks from continuous usage. Fish oils combine well with the other sex boosters discussed in this book.

10. Ginseng

Renowned Asian Energizer

Traditional Chinese herbalists have, for centuries, recommended ginseng to improve vitality and sexual wellness for both sexes. In China, Japan, and Korea, ginseng is commonly included in various herbal products used for the treatment of sexual dysfunction.

There are several varieties of ginseng sold over-the-counter; Asian (Chinese and Korean) ginseng (*Panax ginseng*), American ginseng (*Panax quinquefolius*), and Siberian ginseng (*Eleutherococcus Chinensis*) are the most common. Technically, Siberian ginseng does not belong in the same genus as Asian or American ginseng and does not contain the same substances. As a rule, Chinese ginseng is more stimulating and raises body temperature, while American ginseng is less heating and stimulating. Hundreds of ginseng products are available over-the-counter in varying dosages, forms, and combinations and each of these products may provide a different effect.

WHAT THE RESEARCH SAYS

Korean red ginseng seems to be an effective treatment for erectile dysfunction, according to the results of a small study from Korea. A team at the University of Ulsan and the Korea Ginseng and Tobacco Research Institute in Seoul evaluated Korean red ginseng in forty-five men with erectile dysfunction. The men were randomly assigned to take either 900 mg of ginseng or an inactive placebo pill three times a day.

Eight weeks into the study, the men were taken off the treatment for two weeks, after which they switched treatments for the next eight weeks. Neither the researchers nor the participants knew which pill, ginseng or placebo, the men were taking until after the study was completed.

Reported scores for erectile function, sexual desire, and satisfaction during intercourse were higher when the men were taking ginseng than when they were on the placebo. While they were taking ginseng, 60% of men said that their erections improved, compared to 20% while taking placebo. "Considering that some patients with erectile dysfunction are reluctant to depend on a drug to achieve erection, Korean red ginseng could be used as an alternative remedy," the researchers conclude. A number of studies executed over the years indicate that ginseng has a favorable effect on memory and mood, reaction time, and general quality of life.

HOW IT WORKS

The roots of Chinese and American ginseng contain several saponins named ginsenosides that are believed to contribute to their properties. Saponins are interesting natural compounds found in many plants, herbs, roots, and beans. They are used in traditional Chinese medicine to improve stamina and combat fatigue and stress. Saponins have potential in the prevention and treatment of diseases of the heart and circulatory system. For instance, they inhibit the formation of lipid peroxides (fat oxidation) in cardiac muscle and in the liver. Saponins also influence the function of enzymes; decrease blood coagulation, cholesterol, and sugar levels in the blood; and stimulate the immune system. Some saponins may even have anti-tumor properties.

Recent studies in laboratory animals have shown that both the Asian and American forms of ginseng enhance libido and copulatory performance. These effects of ginseng may not be due to changes in hormone secretion, but to the direct effects of ginseng, or its ginsenoside components, on the central nervous system and gonadal tissues. There is good evidence that ginsenosides can facilitate penile erection by directly inducing the vasodilatation and relaxation of penile corpus cavernosa. Moreover, the effects of ginseng on the corpus cavernosa appear to be mediated by the release of nitric oxide from endothelial cells and from nerves that surround the vessels. Treatment with American ginseng also affects the central nervous system and has been shown to significantly alter the activity of hypothalamic catecholamines, such as dopamine and norephinephrine, involved in the facilitation of copulatory behavior and hormone secretion. According to recent findings, ginseng treatment decreases prolactin secretion, which also suggests a direct effect of ginseng at the level of the pituitary gland. High levels of prolactin inhibit libido.

Studies have sometimes provided contradictory results, perhaps because the ginsenoside content of ginseng root or root extracts can differ depending on the species, method of extraction, subsequent treatment, or even the season of collection.

MY EXPERIENCE

The sexual effects from ginseng are subtle but definitely present. I have tried Asian ginseng on numerous occasions. Most of my trials have been with ginseng root powder at a dosage ranging from 500 to 1,000 mg. I notice an enhancement in alertness, motivation, focus, and mood, along with a mild sexual stimulation. The effects seem to improve on subsequent days of use. I find high doses tend to cause anxiety and interfere with my sleep.

REPORTS FROM PATIENTS

Most patients who take ginseng notice an improvement in energy, vitality, well-being, and mental clarity. About one-third of my patients report an enhancement in sexual interest and performance. It takes several days for the full effects to be noticed.

Harry, a 46-year-old actor, says, "I found that Korean red ginseng was very helpful in making erections last longer. I noticed the effects the third week."

Amber, a 41-year-old graphic artist, says, "I took ginseng for fatigue for a period of three weeks. I felt really better emotionally and had increased energy and sexual vitality. Then I started feeling overly stimulated and had a bad case of insomnia."

CAUTIONS AND SIDE EFFECTS

Insomnia is a common side effect from ginseng overuse, particularly from Asian ginseng—especially when it's combined in high doses with other herbs or nutrients that cause alertness. There are infrequent reports of other side effects, including nervousness and skin eruptions. Individuals with high blood pressure and heart disorders may be prone to heart rhythm irregularities while taking high doses of this sex booster. Therefore, medical consultation is advised for anyone with a chronic medical condition before taking high doses of ginseng, or simply even before taking the supplement for prolonged periods.

DOSAGE AND AVAILABILITY

Countless varieties and dosages of ginseng are available, including dried root, tincture, powder, or liquid extract. One option is to try a product, in capsule form, which has a standardized extract of 3 to 7% ginsenosides. Use 100 mg of this extract in the morning a few times per week. You may require 500 to 2,000 mg of crude extracts to feel the effects of ginseng.

It is difficult to give precise dosage instructions for the various forms of ginseng sold in stores, since there are literally hundreds of vitamin companies who sell ginseng in a variety of doses and forms. The best advice is to purchase a couple products and try them out, beginning with the lowest dose recommended on the label. It would be best to cycle the use of ginseng, since taking breaks will minimize any potential side effects. For instance, you can take it for two or three weeks and then stop taking it for a few weeks.

Many people who take ginseng find this herb to be a good overall energizer and a subtle, yet pleasant, sexual stimulant. Due to the tremendous variety of products sold, it is difficult to give definite dosage recommendations. I would certainly recommend trying a few variations to see which produce the desired effect.

When you shop for ginseng, you will often find it combined with other sex-boosting herbs and supplements. Since ginseng is one of the most popular herbs currently sold, it has found its way into numerous products. Check the individual labels to see how much ginseng has been added. If you are sensitive to herbs, and find that ginseng has a stimulating effect on you, make sure to start with a lower dose. You may have to take half of a capsule or tablet. In the past, ginseng was one of the best known herbal sex boosters; however, over the years, other herbs have begun to take the spotlight, including yohimbe, tribulus, maca, muira puama, and horny goat weed. For more information on these substances, continue reading this book.

11. Horny Goat Weed

Will it Make You Horny, Too?

Horny goat weed (*Epimedium*) is a pungent ornamental herb found in Asia and the Mediterranean. The Chinese call it Yin Yang Huo, which loosely means "licentious goat plant." Legend has it that the name came from a herder who noticed his goats becoming more sexually active after eating the plant. Supplement companies have adopted the provocative name by which it is known in the United States.

The plant was named *epimedium* because it is similar to a plant found in the ancient Asian kingdom of Media, now a part of Iran. *Epimedium* is a genus of many related plant species that are used for medicinal purposes, including *Epimedium sagittatum*, *Epimedium brevicornum*, and *Epimedium koreanum*. Although this herb has a history of traditional use for the treatment of disorders of the kidneys, joints, and liver, its principle use is as an aphrodisiac and to combat fatigue.

WHAT THE RESEARCH SAYS

Very little research has been published in the Western medical literature regarding this plant. One Chinese study investigated the therapeutic effect of *Epimedium sagittatum* (ES) on twenty-two patients with chronic renal failure on hemodialysis. Twelve patients with hemodialysis were served as controls and received placebos. The subjects reported that ES had a sex-enhancing effect and improved their quality of life.

HOW IT WORKS

The exact way in which horny goat weed works remains unclear. Animal studies have shown that it may influence levels of neurotransmitters such as norepinephrine, serotonin, and dopamine. The leaves of horny goat weed contain a variety of flavonoids, icariin, sterols, and an alkaloid called magnaflorine. Flavonoids are thought to enhance nitric oxide formation, which leads to better erections. It is quite likely that horny goat weed positively influences several aspects of human sexual biochemistry.

MY EXPERIENCE

I took five tablets a day of a horny goat weed product. Each tablet contained 500 mg of *Epimedium sagittatum* leaf extract standardized to 10% icariin. I didn't notice much the first two days of use, but on the third day, my general interest in having sex was enhanced. Also, I found many more women to be desirable. These women were of varying appearance, including some that I usually would not find appealing or attractive.

REPORTS FROM PATIENTS

Bill, who is 45, says, "I like horny goat weed, although I find that it takes several days to notice the effects, and I need to take at least two grams per day. My general interest in having sex is enhanced, so I guess I would say that it gives me a higher libido."

Cathy, who is 41, notices the effects of horny goat weed from taking lower doses. "I take one gram per day in the morning on a regular basis, and I try to take a week-long break each month. Horny goat weed has made my sex drive come somewhat closer to my boyfriend's horniness!"

CAUTIONS AND SIDE EFFECTS

No major side effects have yet been discovered. However, in very high doses, horny goat weed may have a stimulatory effect and may also cause sweating or a rise in body temperature.

DOSAGE AND AVAILABILITY

The ideal dosage of horny goat weed is not known, but may range from 1 to 3 g per day. Capsules or tablets are sold in various doses, ranging from 250 to 500 mg. Some products are standardized to a flavonoid called icariin, which has been found to be a strong antioxidant. Not enough research has been done on humans to know whether this standardization to icariin is necessary or desirable.

Horny goat weed is, in fact, likely to make you horny! Most users will notice a mild to moderate sexual effect on the third or fourth day of use. This herb could well be combined with many of the other herbs and nutrients discussed in this book, such as maca, tribulus, ginseng, and others. Since so little is known about horny goat weed, it is difficult to state how long it can be safely taken. Therefore, taking occasional breaks from use is always a good idea until more human research becomes available.

12. Maca

Erotic Incan Herb From the High Andes

Maca (*Lepidium meyenii*) is a root-like vegetable shaped like a radish. It grows in the harsh climate of the Andes Mountains in South America at elevations from 11,000 up to 15,000 feet. Maca is traditionally used in the Andean region for its supposed aphrodisiac and fertility-enhancing properties.

WHAT THE RESEARCH SAYS

In one study, researchers fed high dosages of maca extracts to male mice. As a result, the frequency with which they coupled with female mice tripled. In rats with erectile dysfunction, the time needed between successive couplings was reduced by half.

A human study produced findings similar to those from the rodent one. Researchers at the Universidad Peruana Cayetano Heredia, in Lima, Peru, performed a twelve-week double-blind, randomized trial in which active treatment with different doses of maca was compared with placebo. Men aged 21-56 years received 3 g of maca on a daily basis. An improvement in sexual desire was observed after eight weeks of treatment. Serum testosterone and estradiol levels were not different in men treated with maca than in those treated with placebo, indicating that maca did not have a significant effect on blood hormone levels.

Another study was designed to determine the effect of a four-month oral treatment with maca on seminal fluid analysis in normal adult men aged 24-44 years. Nine men received tablets of maca (1,500 or 3,000 mg per day) for four months. Blood luteinizing hormone, follicle-stimulating hormone, prolactin, testosterone, and estradiol levels were measured before and after treatment. Treatment with maca resulted in the increase of seminal volume, sperm count per ejaculation, and sperm motility. Hormone levels in the blood were not altered.

HOW IT WORKS

Maca contains sterols, uridine, malic acid, macamides, lepidiline A, lepidiline B, and glucosinolates. Many of the compounds in maca have an effect on the central nervous system. The way in which maca works is presently not well understood—but seems to be independent of a significant hormonal effect, since preliminary studies show maca does not influence blood levels of hormones.

MY EXPERIENCE

Within a few hours of taking a high dose of maca, such as four grams, I notice an increase in energy and a sense of well-being. I have found maca to be a mild sex booster at a dose of three grams taken daily for a week.

REPORTS FROM PATIENTS

"The most obvious result from taking maca that I notice is a mild sense of well-being and more vitality," says Debra, who is 52. "Although I sense a slight increase in libido, it's not as pronounced as yohimbe, which I've also tried. I normally take one gram a day."

Peter, who is 39, reports, "There is little doubt that maca gives me more energy and more motivation to do things without postponing. For me, the sexual effects are mild, and in some ways they are similar to ginseng. I normally take one gram a day for a week each month."

CAUTIONS AND SIDE EFFECTS

There have not been any reports of side effects from maca in the medical literature. However, this sex booster does not have a long history of use in North America.

DOSAGE AND AVAILABILITY

Maca is available in capsule form most commonly containing 500 mg of the root. Most users should notice an effect after taking two grams a day for a period of two or three days. As with most of the herbs and supplements discussed in this book, it would be best to cycle the use of maca by taking it for one or two weeks, followed by one or two weeks off. Cycling in such a way will minimize any potential side effects.

Maca seems destined to become more popular with time since human studies indicate that it is a true herbal sex booster. The actions of this Andean aphrodisiac seem more geared towards enhancing libido than just aiding erections. Maca can certainly be combined with other sex-boosting herbs and supplements, and you will find many sexually oriented products on the market that combine maca with several other ingredients.

13. Muira Puama

Brazilian Jungle Passion

Muira puama, also called "potency wood," is a small tree native to the Brazilian Amazon. The tree can reach up to fifteen feet in height. The bark and roots are the primary parts of the plant that are used. Indigenous peoples use muira puama (MP) for the treatment of sexual dysfunction, fatigue, neuromuscular problems, and rheumatism. Muira puama's botanical name is *Ptychopetalum olacoides*, and it is sometimes also referred to as "marapuama."

WHAT THE RESEARCH SAYS

In 1990, at the Institute of Sexology in Paris, France, researchers performed a clinical study with 262 patients complaining of lack of sexual desire. The results demonstrated MP extract to be effective. Within two weeks, at a daily dose of 1 to 1.5 grams of the 4:1 extract, 62% of patients with loss of libido claimed that the treatment was helpful. A 4:1 extract indicates that the active ingredients are concentrated, which makes the muira puama more potent. Although I found this study mentioned all over the internet, I could not find a Medline mention that it had been published in a reliable medical journal.

In 2000, researchers at the Institute of Sexology published another study. The effectiveness of an herbal formulation of MP and Ginkgo biloba was assessed in 202 healthy women affected by low sex drive. Various aspects of their sex life were rated before and after one month of treatment. Statistically significant improvements occurred in sexual intercourse and sexual fantasies, as well as in satisfaction with sex life, intensity of sexual desires, ability to reach orgasm, and intensity of orgasm. Reported tolerability was good.

HOW IT WORKS

The root and bark of muira puama are rich in free long-chain fatty acids, essential oils, plant sterols, coumarin, lupeol, and a new alkaloid named "muirapuamine." Because of its various constituents, it is difficult to pinpoint the exact chemicals in MP that are responsible for its sex-boosting effects. One study in rabbits indicates that MP has the ability to relax the corpus cavernosa of the penis, thus allowing for engorgement.

MY EXPERIENCE

I used muira puama bark in capsule form, each of which contained 250 mg. I took six capsules the first day and noticed within hours feeling more alert, more talkative, and a mild enhancement in visual clarity and libido.

The next day I took eight capsules, totaling 2 g of the MP bark. I definitely noticed having more energy, without feeling stimulated. The experience was quite pleasant. On the third day, I again took 2 g and the effects were similar. I also noticed that I had a stronger interest in having sex and more frequent sexual thoughts.

REPORTS FROM PATIENTS

At least three-quarters of my patients find muira puama to be a helpful sex booster.

James, 48, says, "MP definitely helps my libido, and I notice the effects within four days. I also find it to be a mood enhancer, helping me deal with life's emotional events easier."

Tony, a 44-year-old dentist, reports, "I took MP for one week and noticed that in the mornings my erections were lasting longer. I use an alcoholic tincture. The bottle is a 2 oz container and I use about twenty-five drops in a glass of water. I'm also starting to feel more sensual with a stronger desire."

Cindy, a 34-year-old writer, says, "I have had difficulty feeling aroused since my psychiatrist put me on Prozac. I started MP liquid extract and within two weeks my libido is coming back, although not as much as before Prozac."

David, a 39-year-old therapist, says, "I took one gram of MP for two days. I didn't notice anything the first two days, however, when I awoke the third day, my libido was definitely higher. I was still in bed, and unfortunately my wife had already left for work."

CAUTIONS AND SIDE EFFECTS

There is not enough research available on muira puama to know about any potential long-term side effects. However, high doses of MP may cause insomnia.

DOSAGE AND AVAILABILITY

MP bark is available in capsules containing from 250 to 500 mg, and in a concentrated liquid extract. A range of 500 mg to 2 g of the capsules, or 1 to 2 ml of MP liquid extract taken daily should lead to positive results within a few days.

Muira puama is a reliable sex booster for both men and women. It is not as powerful in inducing erections as yohimbe, however, it is gentler and quite pleasant, providing an enhancement in well-being and visual clarity. MP has historically been combined with catuaba. Some indigenous peoples place the barks of MP and catuaba in a glass of water and drink the resulting infusion the next morning. I like MP because it increases the sensitivity of skin and sexual organs, along with enhancing libido and mood. Try it for at least two weeks before moving on to another sex-boosting supplement.

14. NADH

The Dopamine Connection

You might remember, in your high school biology class, learning about the Krebs cycle and how energy in the form of ATP is derived from sugars, amino acids, and fats. Nicotinamide adenine dinucleotide (NADH) is a coenzyme that helps in this complicated process of energy extraction. NADH is normally found in meat, fish, and poultry. The content of NADH in fruits and vegetables is negligible. I never thought that NADH would one day be available as a supplement, but it was introduced to the health industry as such in the mid 1990s. NADH is actually made of niacin or nicotinamide, one of the B vitamins also known as B3, attached to a coenzyme called adenine dinucleotide; hence the name nicotinamide adenine dinucleotide.

WHAT THE RESEARCH SAYS

A small number of short-term studies show NADH has slight to moderate benefits in the treatment of depression, jet lag, and Parkinson's disease, but does not have a positive effect on those people with Alzheimer's disease. An eight-week double-blind study done at Georgetown University Medical Center found that some patients with chronic fatigue syndrome benefited from taking NADH at a daily dose of 10 mg. However, long-term studies are required to determine whether the benefits from taking NADH daily continue over time or if tolerance develops.

There have not been any studies that have focused on the effect of supplemental NADH on the human sexual response.

HOW IT WORKS

One of the functions of NADH is helping to convert the amino acid tyrosine into the vital brain chemical dopamine. Dopamine is an important neurotransmitter involved in mood, energy, sex drive, and muscle movement. (See Chapter 1 for more information on dopamine.) Tyrosine hydroxylase is the rate-limiting enzyme—or that which is in shortest supply—in the synthesis of dopamine from tyrosine. NADH helps the function of this enzyme, and hence more dopamine can be produced. NADH also regenerates the antioxidant glutathione, which provides general health benefits.

MY EXPERIENCE

I have taken NADH on numerous occasions. Within an hour or two after swallowing a pill on an empty stomach in the morning, I notice an increase in alertness, well-being, visual clarity, and sexual interest. The effects last most of the day. I also find that my interest in sex continues the day after taking NADH. If I take more than 10 mg, even in the morning, I find that I am still alert at bedtime and not able to get a deep sleep. I also seem to develop a tolerance to NADH if I take it regularly; I just don't notice the effects as much after a while.

REPORTS FROM PATIENTS

Most people who take NADH notice an enhancement in energy, mood, and alertness.

Alice, age 52, says, "I have taken 10 mg NADH daily for one month and it makes a huge difference to my energy level. Not that I take a pill and then feel like I'm on speed, but more like I take a pill in the morning and that evening I look back at what I've done for that day and realize how much I've accomplished. I've noticed that

I only garden on those days I take NADH. My husband tells me that I'm more responsive to him sexually when I take this supplement."

Mark, a 56-year-old accountant, says, "I take 2.5 mg of NADH three times a week. My brain is working again. I can think clearer and sharper, and I have a stronger libido."

Shirley, age 44, reports, "NADH makes me more alert and provides a sense of well-being. I find myself thinking about sex more often."

Development of tolerance seems to be an issue with some individuals. I have come across several people who thought that the effects from NADH did not continue for very long. Here are three reports:

"I tried NADH for a while and at first it was wonderful. However, after about a month or two I didn't notice the energy boost anymore."

"I've been taking 10 mg of NADH for about eight months. It helped me noticeably in the beginning. Now I find that if I miss a few days, I don't notice any change."

"I have been taking 5 mg of NADH for about a month. The first week I felt better than I had in years, but since then, the effect seems to be fading."

CAUTIONS AND SIDE EFFECTS

There have not been reports of any major side effects with NADH, however a few people have noticed mild insomnia, stomach pains, agitation, and mood swings. Sleepiness or yawning can occur for brief moments throughout the day. Be careful when using multiple supplements that increase energy, since their effects can be additive and lead to overstimulation.

DOSAGE AND AVAILABILITY

NADH is widely available from different manufacturers. Most of the NADH pills come in dosages of 2.5, 5, and 10 mg. There is also a sublingual version available. Individually sealed airtight pills are a good option. NADH is generally more expensive than many of the other supplements discussed in this book. Take NADH on an empty stomach with a glass of water at least twenty minutes before breakfast, or before lunch.

NADH is a supplement helpful for boosting your energy level, sense of alertness, and libido. If you plan to take NADH on a regular basis, limit your frequency to no more than twice a week. Until we learn more about NADH, I do not recommend its use on a daily basis for prolonged periods. For a quick effect, you may consider the 10 mg pills, however, you may do well with 2.5 or 5 mg taken over several days. The lower doses are likely to cause fewer side effects. You may choose to take NADH for a few days and then take a break for several weeks and try a different natural sex booster during that time.

15. Pregnenolone
Hormone of High Sensation

Most people, including many in the medical profession, have not heard of pregnenolone (preg), yet this hormone has very interesting properties. When used appropriately, preg can provide a peaceful sense of well-being; enhanced alertness and awareness; heightened visual and auditory perception; better memory, verbal fluency, and concentration; and most importantly for the purposes of this book, a stronger sex drive with enhanced genital sensation. However, preg is a powerful hormone with potentially serious side effects if misused.

WHAT THE RESEARCH SAYS

Preg was first discovered in 1934, and the results of many human studies done in the 1940s showed that this hormone could combat fatigue, ease arthritic pain, and enhance thinking ability. However, in the 1940s, around the same time as the research on preg, cortisone, another closely related hormone, was being tested. Cortisone soon took the spotlight and researchers basically forgot about doing studies on preg. I am not aware of any human research that directly evaluates the sex-boosting effect of pregnenolone.

HOW IT WORKS

Preg is a steroid hormone made from cholesterol in the adrenal glands, ovaries, and testicles, but it can also be made in other tissues, including the brain. In the brain and nervous system, preg is identified as a neurosteroid and is involved in remodeling nerve cells and influencing the action of neurotransmitters.

I call preg the "grandmother of all the adrenal hormones" since the body uses it to convert into DHEA, progesterone, and at least one hundred different steroid hormones. When you swallow a preg pill, it makes its way into the bloodstream and then travels around to the rest of the body, entering a variety of tissues and cells. Preg is then converted into DHEA, which, in turn, has the ability to convert into androstenedione, testosterone, and estrogens. Preg can also convert into progesterone, which is one of the qualities that makes it different from DHEA.

Therefore, one way that preg could enhance sexual enjoyment is through its conversion into androgens. It has also been shown in animal studies that preg influences acetylcholine levels (and perhaps also dopamine), which could also explain its beneficial effects. You may remember from Chapter 1 that acetylcholine contributes to the engorgement of the genital organs, and dopamine has a significant effect on sexual desire.

MY EXPERIENCE

I have taken preg on numerous occasions in dosages ranging from 2 to 50 mg. Preg improves my visual and auditory perception, and also provides a sense of well-being. After several days of taking 5 to 10 mg, I notice an increase in my sex drive with an enhancement of skin sensation. I have not noticed a significant effect on erections.

I have also experienced side effects from preg including headaches, acne, insomnia, irritability, and heart palpitations, when on dosages greater than 20 mg. I only use preg as a sex booster once or twice a month.

REPORTS FROM PATIENTS

Most patients report that this hormone enhances alertness and arousal, and has a profound effect on memory and awareness. At least one-third notice an enhancement in visual perception. About one-half find an increase in sexual enjoyment, but the sexual effects do not seem as consistent as that of DHEA.

Joanne, a 44-year-old hairdresser with a lagging sex drive, says, "I heard about pregnenolone from a friend who had tried it for PMS. She mentioned that her vision had improved the very day she took it. I tried 10 mg for three days in a row starting on Thursday morning. On Saturday evening, my husband and I were in the living room and he started touching me on my belly and breasts. It felt much more sensual than his normal touch."

Gary, who is 51, says, "Within a few days of taking 10 mg of pregnenolone, I realized that women had become much more attractive to me. I realized that there was a certain magic in the female form that had gradually escaped from me over the years, without me realizing this loss. I definitely believe that this hormone enhanced my libido."

CAUTIONS AND SIDE EFFECTS

High doses of preg can lead to androgenic side effects similar to those from DHEA, including acne and accelerated hair loss (with prolonged use). Irritability, aggressiveness, insomnia, anxiety, headaches, and menstrual irregularities are also reported. Heart palpitations can occur in dosages greater than 20 mg, or even at 5 mg in individuals prone to irregular heart rhythms. Since preg enhances nerve sensation, I have had some patients report that when they took this hormone while having nerve-related pain, such as sciatica, their pain increased. I am still not sure if there is a connection, but it is possible.

DOSAGE AND AVAILABILITY

Preg pills and sublingual tablets are sold in dosages starting at 5 mg upwards to 50 mg. It would be prudent if companies voluntarily restricted their maximum dosage of preg to no more than 10 mg per tablet in order to avoid or minimize some of the possible side effects, such as skipped heartbeats.

Some people notice the effects from preg within hours, but it often takes several days to notice the full impact. One option is to take 5 mg in the morning and around noon for a few days, and then stop. If you do plan to use preg regularly, it is best to limit your frequency to a few days per month. It may be difficult to find preg in smaller doses such as 5 mg; hence you may consider purchasing the 10 mg capsules or tablets and taking half the amount.

Preg and DHEA have overlapping functions; therefore, if you plan to add preg to your DHEA regimen, reduce your dosage of DHEA by the appropriate corresponding milligram amount. The same applies to androstenedione. Preg is best taken in the morning, or no later than noon.

Preg is a fascinating hormone with very pleasant effects. There is still a great deal we need to learn about preg's potential. Caution is advised until we learn more. Keep your dosage level to a minimum, and when you learn to use this hormone appropriately, you will really appreciate the overall sensual enhancement it provides. Medical supervision is recommended when considering the use of hormones, particularly if you intend to use them for longer than a few days.

16. Tongkat Ali

Exotic Asian Aphrodisiac

Tongkat ali (*Eurycoma longifolia jack*) is a tree found in the jungles throughout Malaysia and Southeast Asia. It is commonly known as "tongkat ali" in Malaysia and Singapore, and "pasak bumi" in Indonesia. The tree can grow up to twelve meters in height. Indigenous peoples consider every part of the tree as medicine and the roots have been used as a tonic, to treat malaria, and as an aphrodisiac.

In the old days, the roots had to be brewed for many long hours to get a bitter extract. Now, tongkat ali, which literally means Ali's cane or stick, is conveniently packed in pill or tea-bag form and mixed with regular coffee or tea. Tongkat ali coffee and tea are now sold in Malaysia's roadside peddler stands, supermarkets, and even at eateries in posh hotels. In the United States, tongkat ali is being promoted by some herbal companies under the popular alternative name of "Long Jack."

WHAT THE RESEARCH SAYS

Over the past few years, there have been quite a number of studies that have shown tongkat ali to have sex-boosting properties. The effects of tongkat ali were studied on the libido of male rats after dosing them with up to 800 mg per kilogram of body weight twice daily for ten days. Results showed that tongkat ali produced a dose-dependent increase in mounting frequency, that is, the number of times the male rats tried to mount the female rats increased as the dose given to the rats increased. In addition, the rats displayed more frequent and vigorous licking and anogenital sniffing towards the receptive females. Furthermore, the rats dosed with tongkat ali spent more time grooming their genitals compared to the rats who were not given the plant. Genital grooming may be interpreted as masturbation. The researchers noticed another interesting finding; while the rats who had not received the plant showed normal behavior within the cage, such as exploration and climbing the cage wall, the rats given tongkat ali stayed around the females instead of exploring the cage. Tongkat ali also increased the frequency of the rats' erections. Interestingly, scientists have found that, in addition to its sex-enhancing effects, compounds within this plant have anti-malarial properties.

HOW IT WORKS

Very little is known regarding the way in which tongkat ali works. Recent studies indicate that the root contains several compounds, including beta-carboline alkaloids and quassinoid-type glycosides. How these compounds, and others in tongkat ali, influence the human sexual response is not clearly understood at this time. I have read promotional material by some vitamin companies regarding tongkat ali, which states that it enhances the production of testosterone; however, I have not been able to conclusively confirm this claim through a Medline search.

MY EXPERIENCE

I have taken both the raw powder and extracts of tongkat ali. After several weeks of trying this plant in various doses and during different times of the day, I discovered that tongkat ali is best taken in the early morning. This is because the effects start within a few hours and last all day, and if a high dose is taken, insomnia can occur. Tongkat ali's influence on the body can last a long time, sometimes up to two days.

I find that taking 500 to 1,000 mg of the raw powder works well for me. There are now several extracts of tongkat ali that are being marketed. Some of these extracts include 20:1 and 100:1—meaning that, since the active ingredients are concentrated, a 100:1 extract is thought to be one-hundred times as powerful per weight as an equivalent amount of plain powder, although there is no research yet to give us a clear answer on exactly how many times more potent the 100:1 extract is compared to the raw powder. I find that a small dose of the 100:1 extract, such as 40 to 100 mg, is effective, leading to increased libido, more frequent sexual thoughts, more energy, and a longer lasting erection. Sometimes I also notice more alertness and genital sensitivity, clearer vision, plus a slight improvement in well-being. One morning, after taking tongkat ali, I went on a bike ride and then had lunch with a friend. I found myself more energetic, talkative, and in an upbeat mood.

A common side effect that I noticed from high doses of tongkat ali is insomnia. This happens even if I take it in the morning. Another side effect on high doses may be a feeling of restlessness, and increased body temperature.

REPORTS FROM PATIENTS

Janet, 35, took one capsule containing 60 mg of a 100:1 extract at 5:00 PM. She says, "Within two hours I became more alert and the first thing I noticed was that my nipples were more sensitive. Normally I have a cigarette after sex, but this time I didn't feel the urge to have one. I did have trouble sleeping overnight since I felt more alert than usual."

Art, a 47-year-old accountant, found tongkat ali to be helpful in improving his sexual relationship with his wife. He says, "My sex life had lost passion. After twenty years of marriage, my wife and I had basically settled into a lackluster once-a-week on Saturday night routine. I took 1,000 mg of tongkat ali powder on a Wednesday morning and by midday, while at work, I started thinking about my wife. I couldn't wait to get home that evening. She was quite surprised when I came home with a big smile and started caressing her in a sensual way."

CAUTIONS AND SIDE EFFECTS

High doses could lead to overstimulation and insomnia, a feeling of restlessness or irritation, and perhaps a slightly higher body temperature, but thus far, in my limited experience, I have not come across any other side effect. We do need to keep in mind, though, that no human trials of any significant length are available to indicate whether this aphrodisiac has long-term harmful effects. For now, it seems quite acceptable to use a small amount of tongkat ali, and to be on the safe side, no more than two or three days a week.

DOSAGE AND AVAILABILITY

Tongkat ali is sold as a root powder, in capsules containing 300 to 700 mg of the root powder. You will also find it in a variety of extracts, ranging up to a 100:1 potency. You may notice different effects from different products, since one cannot assume that extracts from various companies will be similar in potency. Therefore, it is quite difficult to provide accurate dosage recommendations for the extracts. Women are likely to respond to smaller doses, while men may need a higher amount. You will also find products that are labeled Long Jack; this is the same as tongkat ali since companies often use this abbreviation of the scientific name *Eurycoma longifolia jack*. Some manufacturers, particularly in Asia, add this sex booster to energy drinks and coffee.

Tongkat ali works well, however do not expect it to be effective right away, such as yohimbe, which works within an hour or two. Tongkat ali, along with yohimbe, is probably one of the most consistently effective herbal sex boosters. I really enjoy my experiences with tongkat ali. If you take it in the morning, you may notice the effects by late afternoon or evening, or even the next day. Insomnia is one of the major shortcomings of tongkat ali, and therefore you may need to experiment with different doses and products to find the amount that works for you without interfering with your deep sleep.

17. Tribulus

Roadside Sex Weed that Works

Tribulus terrestris, also called "puncture vine," is a plant that has been long used around the world for the treatment of various ailments, and popularly claimed to improve sexual function in humans. In Turkey, tribulus terrestris (TT) is commonly used in folk medicine for the treatment of abdominal colic, hypertension, and high cholesterol. In Europe, the plant has been a part of natural medicine throughout history—as far back as ancient Greece—for the treatment of such varied conditions as headache, nervous disorders, constipation, and sexual dysfunction. In China and India, tribulus terrestris has been celebrated for its beneficial role in liver, kidney, urinary, and cardiovascular remedies.

TT grows naturally in many parts of the world, including the Americas, Australia, Europe, Middle East, and Africa. It is considered a noxious weed, and is found abundantly on roadsides and in vacant lots, with seeds that are sharp and painful to step on. Tribulus terrestris's foliage is toxic to livestock, especially sheep, when consumed in large quantities. The fruits or berries are the parts of the plant most often used in traditional medicine. The composition of the different substances found within TT will likely vary, depending on the part of the world in which the plant grows.

WHAT THE RESEARCH SAYS

Several studies with rodents indicate that tribulus terrestris is helpful as a sex booster. In one study conducted at National University in Singapore, sexual behavior and intracavernous pressure (ICP) measurements were taken in rats to scientifically validate the claim of TT as an aphrodisiac. ICP refers to blood flow into the corpus cavernosa of the penis, the spongy tubes where blood accumulates to cause an erection. The more blood that comes in, the higher the pressure will be inside the corpus cavernosa.

Forty sexually mature male rats were randomly divided into four groups of ten each. Group I served as a control group (they did not receive any TT) and groups II, III, and IV were treated with three different doses of TT extract (2.5, 5, and 10 mg/kg body weight, respectively). The doses were administered orally, once daily for eight weeks. Weight was recorded and the rats from all four groups were subjected to sexual behavior studies with primed females. Various parameters were measured, particularly mounting frequency (MF). MF is the number of times the male rats attempted to mount the female rats. Increases in body weight (by 9%, 23%, and 18% for groups II, III, and IV) and ICP (by 43% and 26% for groups III and IV) were statistically significant compared to the control group. Increases in MF (by 27% for group III and 24% for group IV) were also statistically significant.

The authors of the study conclude, "The weight gain and improvement in sexual behavior parameters observed in rats could be secondary to the androgen-increasing property of TT that was observed in our earlier study on primates. The increase in ICP, which confirms the proerectile aphrodisiac property of TT, could possibly be the result of an increase in androgen and subsequent release of nitric oxide from the nerve endings innervating the corpus cavernosum."

Tribulus terrestris has been studied in China and found to reduce the frequency of angina pectoris in humans. Laboratory studies have also found TT to have anti-microbial and anti-tumor potential. A few studies involving rodents indicate that TT lowers blood pressure, blood sugar, and reduces levels of triglycerides in the blood. I have not seen any substantial evidence that TT enhances athletic performance.

HOW IT WORKS

Tribulus terrestris seems to work by relaxing smooth muscles and increasing blood flow into the corpus cavernosa. The relaxant effect observed is probably due to the increase in the release of nitric oxide from the endothelium (a thin layer of flattened cells that lines blood vessels) and nerve endings. Since TT relaxes smooth muscles, this may account for its benefits in the treatment of abdominal colic.

The fruits of TT contain a number of different substances including saponins, glycosides, flavonoids, alkaloids, resins, tannins, sugars, sterols, and essential oil. Saponins are substances found in soybeans and many other plants and herbs, including ginseng. A saponin is a molecule that has one part that dissolves easily into oil, and one part that dissolves into water, thus producing foam when mixed with water. Research shows that saponins produce many effects in the body, including the lowering of cholesterol, the influencing of hormone levels, and the potential boosting of sexuality.

A frequently recognized substance in TT is protodioscin, which is believed to be one of the active saponin substances within this plant. Upon analysis of different samples of TT, significant differences in the composition of saponins are observed. These differences are due to the origin of each individual plant, and the particular part that is tested. One analysis of products showed considerable variations—ranging from 0.17% to 6.5%—in the level of protodioscin content.

MY EXPERIENCE

One morning, I took three tablets, each containing 750 mg, of TT. I noticed a slight to moderate enhancement in libido and slightly stronger erections later that day. A few days later, I took a total of six pills within a three-hour period in the morning. I definitely noticed feeling more aroused and a boost in my sexual thoughts and desire that afternoon and evening.

REPORTS FROM PATIENTS

John, a 37-year-old who took TT for one week, says, "I noticed that I was a little more sexually aggressive and my girlfriend's body was more exciting to look at and touch."

Leonard, who is 56, says, "Getting an erection has been a struggle for me for quite a while. After four days of taking 1.5 g of TT, I could stay up longer, and I've noticed my penis is making some attempts at spontaneous erections."

Joey, 34, says, "TT does increase my libido and sensation in my penis."

Some women find TT to be beneficial. Carol, who is 45, says, "After taking 1 g of TT for several days, I noticed that I was thinking about sex more often and had a stronger urge to be intimate."

CAUTIONS AND SIDE EFFECTS

No side effects have yet been reported in the medical literature regarding the use of tribulus terrestris. However, little is known about its long-term use in humans.

DOSAGE AND AVAILABILITY

TT is widely available in health and vitamin stores either by itself or, more often, combined with other sex boosters or hormones. Capsules are usually sold containing from 300 to 750 mg of TT. A daily dose of one or two grams is a suggested guideline for taking tribulus terrestris. The use of TT can be cycled, for instance, alternate by taking it for one week and then stop for one week. Taking breaks minimizes any potential side effects that we may not yet be aware of.

Recently, various extracts of TT have become available, such as 20% saponins and 40% saponins, or those listed by the percentage of protodioscin content, but too little is known about these extracts to make any firm recommendations on dosages.

Tribulus terrestris has moderate libido- and erection-enhancing properties. A daily dose of TT could be combined with some of the hormones, such as androstenedione and DHEA. TT can also be combined with other herbs such as catuaba, muira puama, tongkat ali, yohimbe, and others. Preliminary research in rodents indicates this herb can be beneficial in reducing blood lipids—probably due to its saponin content. However, as with most of the sex boosters discussed in this book, TT can not yet be recommended for long-term use since little is known about its effect in humans if ingested for prolonged periods.

18. Yohimbe

Experience the Orgiastic Mating Rituals of the African Bantu

Yohimbe is one of the most popular and effective sex stimulants for both men and women. It is the name of the bark of a tall evergreen tree in western Africa known as *Pausinystalia yohimbe* or *Corynanthe yohimbe*. According to early historical records, Bantu tribes ingested inner bark shavings of the yohimbe tree to sustain them during extended orgiastic mating rituals that would last up to two weeks.

The active ingredient in yohimbe bark is yohimbine. In the 1970s and early '80s, the existing literature on yohimbine often acknowledged that it could facilitate erection but usually claimed that it had no impact on libido. These sources stated that yohimbine was therefore definitely not a real aphrodisiac. Such pronouncements persisted until a widely acclaimed animal study published in 1984 provided strong evidence that yohimbine stimulates libido in rats and thereby qualifies as a true aphrodisiac. Over the next few years, a series of studies were published concerning yohimbine's efficacy in treating male impotence. FDA approval for this indication soon followed, and, after a twenty-year absence, yohimbine reappeared on the roster of drugs that could be dispensed legally by prescription. Currently, several pharmaceutical companies have yohimbine available as a prescription drug to treat erectile dysfunction. However, the popularity of yohimbine has decreased since the introduction of Viagra and similar drugs.

WHAT THE RESEARCH SAYS

Almost all clinical studies to date have been conducted with yohimbine rather than yohimbe bark. Yohimbine has been evaluated in the treatment of sexual dysfunction through many placebo-controlled trials. It does appear to have a therapeutic benefit, particularly in psychological cases of erectile disorder.

In 1977, a German double-blind, placebo-controlled clinical trial of yohimbine hydrochloride included eighty-six patients with erectile dysfunction and without clearly detectable organic or psychological causes. Yohimbine was administered orally in a dosage of 30 mg per day (two 5 mg tablets three times daily) for eight weeks. Patients were seen for follow-up after four weeks of treatment, and for a final visit after the eight weeks. Efficacy evaluation was based on both subjective and objective criteria. Subjective criteria included improvement in sexual desire, sexual satisfaction, frequency of sexual contacts, and quality of erection (penile rigidity) during sexual contact or intercourse. Objective criteria were based on improvement in penile rigidity. Overall, yohimbine was found significantly more effective than placebo in terms of response rate: 71% versus 45%. Yohimbine was well tolerated; only 7% of patients rated tolerability fair or poor, and most adverse experiences were mild. There were no serious negative effects reported.

A combination study evaluating yohimbine and arginine for the treatment of erectile dysfunction was conducted at Hopital Foch, Suresnes, in France. The goal of this double-blind, placebo-controlled, randomized clinical trial was to compare the efficacy and safety of the combination of 6 g of L-arginine and 6 mg of yohimbine, with that of 6 mg of yohimbine alone, and that of placebo alone in thirty-four patients. During each of the two-week crossover periods, the medicines were administered orally, one to two hours before intended sexual intercourse. The results showed that the L-arginine and yohimbine combination is effective in improving erectile function in patients with mild to moderate erectile dysfunction.

Is yohimbine effective in women? A study conducted at the University of Texas at Austin examined the effects of arginine combined with yohimbine on sexual arousal in postmenopausal women with

98

Female Sexual Arousal Disorder. Twenty-four women participated in three treatment sessions in which subjective reports and vaginal sexual responses to erotic stimuli were measured following treatment with either L-arginine (6 g) plus yohimbine (6 mg), yohimbine alone (6 mg), or placebo, using a randomized, double-blind design. Sexual responses were measured at approximately sixty minutes post-drug administration. The combined oral administration of L-arginine and yohimbine substantially increased vaginal pulse amplitude responses to viewing an erotic film at sixty minutes post-drug administration, compared with placebo. The vaginal response was measured with an instrument called a vaginal photoplethysmograph.

HOW IT WORKS

Unlike many of the other herbs discussed in this book whose mechanism of action is not clearly understood, there has been quite a great deal of research regarding yohimbine's physiological properties. Yohimbine acts through the brain and spinal cord, and also has an influence on the peripheral nervous system—the nerves in the body beyond the brain and spinal cord. In the brain, yohimbine stimulates the release of norepinephrine, which increases sexual arousal and body temperature. Peripherally, yohimbine blocks alpha 2-adrenoceptors in the nerves of the genital region. In a non-aroused state, the normal amount of norepinephrine circulating in the bloodstream stimulates alpha 2-adrenoceptors in the blood vessels and corpora cavernosa, which makes erections difficult. Yohimbine blocks the action of norepinephrine on the alpha 2-adrenoceptors in the genital area, thus allowing dilation of blood vessels and the corpora cavernosa. By doing so, blood flow to the penis is increased and engorgement occurs. It is also possible that yohimbine stimulates the dopamine system in the brain, and increases sexual interest. For more details about the role of dopamine, see Chapter 1.

MY EXPERIENCE

Yohimbe definitely works. I notice an enhanced, longer-lasting erection from yohimbe in about an hour and a half after intake. Upon taking higher dosages, such as 300 mg or more, I feel a more pronounced effect on erection, however the side effects are more uncomfortable. I have experienced rapid heart beat with sweating, restlessness, and blurring of vision when ingesting 600 mg. However, on a lower dosage such as 100 to 250 mg, I have not experienced any significant side effects. In addition to improving my erections, yohimbe also enhances my sexual interest and pleasure.

REPORTS FROM PATIENTS

Yohimbe users consistently glow about the positive benefits of taking this substance. The majority of users like this natural sex booster, but some are concerned about the side effects.

One of my patients is Lora, a 42-year-old beautician who took 150 mg of yohimbe shortly after a small lunch. She says, "I went shopping with my boyfriend after lunch for an hour, then we went to my apartment. I noticed that my body was warmer, and I was starting to get in the mood. I initiated some contact and we ended up having a very enjoyable time. I could tell my clitoris was more engorged than normal, and it seemed more sensitive. A few days later, I took two capsules, and the experience was even better. I got in the mood right away and had such an enhanced sensation of my nipples and vagina."

Ken, a 38-year-old accountant, has difficulty with erections when he is under stress, particularly during tax season. He says, "I find 300 mg of yohimbe to be quite effective, with hardly any side effects except for slight sweating. I can stay hard for at least thirty minutes whereas without it I can only maintain an erection for a few minutes before having an embarrassing deflation. My wife now thinks that I find her more appealing since I stay harder longer."

CAUTIONS AND SIDE EFFECTS

Yohimbe can be quite harsh for some people, particularly when high doses are taken. One patient says, "I get quite horny from yohimbe, but I don't like the feeling of anxiety, sweating, and restlessness that it brings on."

Yohimbe should be used cautiously by anyone with a medical condition, especially those with hypertension, heart disease, diabetes, or those taking medicines—particularly tranquilizers, antidepressants, sedatives, antihistamines, and amphetamines or other stimulants, including caffeine. Some of the side effects from doses greater than 300 mg of yohimbe include anxiety, elevated blood pressure, heart rate increase or palpitations, dizziness, headache, tremor, visual disturbances, nausea or abdominal cramps, increased body temperature, and sweating.

Since high doses of yohimbe may cause confusion and disorientation, it should not be taken while operating machinery, driving, or performing hazardous activities. Yohimbe is also not recommended for those who are on psychiatric medicines unless approved by a physician.

DOSAGE AND AVAILABILITY

Yohimbine is a pharmaceutical drug, while yohimbe is sold over-the-counter. Yohimbine, as a prescription drug, is often standardized at about 5 mg per tablet. Most yohimbe sold over-the-counter is in tablet or capsule form containing 200 to 1,000 mg of yohimbe bark. Yohimbe is also available as a tincture, but I have little personal experience with this form. If the product you purchase contains more than 300 mg of yohimbe, consider initially taking a portion of the pill or capsule. Gradually increase the dose to achieve the desired effect. The effects are noticeable within an hour or two.

Yohimbe bark has been reported to contain up to 6% total alkaloids, 10 to 15% of which is yohimbine. One can make a rough estimate of the amount of yohimbine present in a yohimbe product—for instance a capsule that has 300 mg of yohimbe. Assuming there are 6% of alkaloids present in the product, 300 mg of yohimbe would have 18 mg of alkaloids. And if we assume 15% of the alkaloids are yohimbine, then we can estimate about 2.7 mg of yohimbine to be present in a 300 mg capsule or tablet of yohimbe. In contrast, many of the yohimbine products available through a doctor's prescription contain about 5 mg of yohimbine.

In addition to plain yohimbe bark, many products now include extracts of various potencies—including 4% alkaloids, and even 8%, 10%, and 20% as well. The higher the percentage, the more potent the yohimbe, and less of it will be required to achieve the desired effects. However, very little is known regarding the effective dosages of different extracts. There may even be differences between the many product manufacturers. If you are interested in trying yohimbe extracts, start with a small amount and gradually increase to reach the desired effect.

Yohimbe may be used either daily or before planned sexual activity. In my opinion, since yohimbe works rather quickly, it makes sense that it be taken as needed—such as one to three hours before sexual intercourse—rather than taken daily. The effects last several hours.

Yohimbine has been studied quite extensively, and most results show it to be effective in helping with erections, particularly in those whose erectile dysfunction is due to psychological causes. Results of studies have also shown this substance to be quite helpful in women. My clinical experience indicates that yohimbe works quite well. Side effects, particularly nervousness and heart pounding, are the limiting factors in the use of yohimbe in high doses. It is possible to minimize the side effects of yohimbe by taking a low dose such as 300 mg or less, and using it only when needed, as opposed to daily intake.

19. Additional Sex Boosters

Potential Libido Lifts

In addition to the natural sex-boosting herbs, supplements, and hormones that I discuss in this book, there are many others that are historically known or currently promoted as having aphrodisiac properties. In this chapter, I will mention a few herbs that you may come across while you are researching this topic, or that you may see on the label ingredient list of sex-enhancing products. These herbs are included in this chapter, as opposed to the main part of the book, for two major reasons: either there is a scarcity of research evaluating their benefits, or perhaps they do not have a significant immediate sexual effect. Future research will give us a better understanding regarding the role of these herbs as potential aphrodisiacs.

CNIDIUM MONNIERI

Cnidium is a plant that grows in China (and possibly in Oregon) whose seeds have been used in traditional Chinese medicine for skin problems, and as a natural sex booster. It is known in China as *She Chuang Zi*.

Cnidium seed contains several compounds including coumarins, osthol, imperatorin, glucides, and sesquiterpenes (which are thought to be protective of the liver). Preliminary studies show that some of the compounds in cnidium may have antihistamine, anti-itch, anti-fungal, and antibacterial effects, along with having an influence on the pituitary-adrenocortical axis of the brain. Additional studies on rodents indicate that cnidium may improve bone strength. A compound found in cnidium called osthol or osthole was found in rabbits to help relax the corpus cavernosa of the penis, which could improve blood flow and facilitate erections. I have not come across human trials regarding the clinical use of cnidium for sex-boosting purposes.

I have only had the opportunity to try cnidium on two separate occasions, each at a dose of 600 mg. I obtained the cnidium powder from a bulk herbal supplier. Each time, I noticed a slight enhanced interest in sex within a few hours, with thoughts occasionally returning to sexuality throughout the day. I also noticed a mild improvement in alertness and a slightly improved clarity in vision. I have not had a chance to have patients or friends try this herb.

Cnidium is not readily available by itself in stores; however, you may occasionally come across it as one of the ingredients listed in libido-boosting products. There is very little known about cnidium in the Western medical literature, and therefore no firm guidelines as to its use can be provided at this time.

DAMIANA

Damiana is a small shrub with aromatic leaves that is often found growing on dry, sunny, rocky hillsides in southern Texas, Mexico, and Central America. Damiana leaves have been used as an aphrodisiac and to boost sexual potency by the native peoples of Mexico, including the Mayan Indians. The two species used in herbal healing, both of which are referred to as damiana, are *Turnera aphrodisiaca* and *Turnera diffusa.*

Damiana contains flavones, gonzalitosin, arbutin, tannin, and damianin (a brown bitter substance). The libido-boosting power of damiana has not been tested in humans, although a liquor made from the leaves has long been used as an aphrodisiac in Mexico. In animal studies, extracts of damiana sped up the mating behavior of sexually sluggish, or impotent, male rats. The extracts had no effect on sexually potent rats.

I have only tried damiana once. I took 2 g of damiana for three days but did not notice much of an effect. Perhaps the amount I took was too little, or I did not take it for a long enough time period. I have also had one of my patients try 2 g of damiana for three days in a row, but she did not notice much of a libido boost either.

Damiana appears to be a safe herb. It is available as a tincture and in capsules commonly containing 500 mg of damiana powder. I have had only limited experience with this herb, but I suspect it is not a powerful aphrodisiac when used by itself. Although the sex-boosting effects of damiana may be appreciated by some users, I see its role in combination with more effective sex-boosting herbs as muira puama, horny goat weed, tribulus, and yohimbe.

DEER ANTLER VELVET

A 2,000-year-old scroll discovered in a tomb in Hunan Province, China, lists dozens of different diseases that could be treated with deer velvet. The sixteenth century *Materia Medica*, a standard text of Chinese herbalists, lists deer velvet as one of the most highly prized natural medicinal substances.

Deer antler is named after the soft, velvet-like covering that deer antlers have before they turn bony. Antlers are organs of bone that regenerate each year from the heads of male deer. In addition to bone, support tissues such as nerves also regenerate. Nerves grow up to 1 cm each day. Antler velvet contains many substances including amino acids, minerals, proteins, anti-inflammatory peptides, hormones, gangliosides and glycosaminoglycans, and Insulin-like growth factor 1. The composition of velvet supplements depends on the diet of the deer, climate, time of year, age of the stag, and the various concentrations of substances in the different parts of the antler velvet itself.

Research studies with deer antler velvet in relation to sexual function are quite limited. A Russian study with pantocrin, an extract from deer antler velvet, showed the extract to stimulate sexual behavior in rodents more than ginseng. Another study showed velvet to have anti-inflammatory properties and to be potentially helpful in the treatment of rheumatoid arthritis. No toxic effects have been found with the use of deer velvet when tested in rodents.

I have only come across one thorough study regarding the influence of deer velvet on the human sexual response. Researchers at the University of Waikato, Hamilton, New Zealand, investigated sexual function in men during a twelve-week double-blind, placebo-controlled trial of deer velvet. Thirty-two male participants, aged 45-65 years, and their partners, were randomly assigned to either the deer velvet or placebo study group. The males took capsules containing ground deer velvet or the placebo every day for twelve weeks. Blood tests at baseline, and the end of the study, determined the levels of sex-related hormones in male participants. There were no significant hormonal changes from baseline to the end of the study in either group of men. The investigators concluded that, in normal males, there was no advantage in taking deer velvet to enhance sexual function.

Deer antler velvet is sold in a variety of dosages, most commonly 250 mg. Since deer antler velvet products are available from many countries and regions, one can expect variations in composition between different products. I have not yet had any personal experience with deer antler velvet, and I cannot provide any recommendations on its use.

GINKGO

Extracts from the leaves of the ginkgo biloba tree have been used therapeutically in China for millennia. The primary indications for ginkgo are age-related mental decline and Alzheimer's disease. Ginkgo is also helpful in the treatment of macular degeneration.

I have not come across any research directly examining the effects of ginkgo on libido. There was a study published which showed that ginkgo, when given to patients who were on SSRI antidepressants such as Prozac, was able to reverse some of the medication-induced sexual dysfunction. However, results of a later study did not find ginkgo helpful in reversing the libido-busting side effects of such antidepressants.

Ginkgo improves blood flow and oxygenation of tissues. The active ingredients in ginkgo act as antioxidants, prevent red blood cells and platelets from aggregating to form clots, and improve circulation in tiny blood vessels by inducing relaxation of the muscles surrounding blood vessels. These properties may be of importance to the men and women who have sexual dysfunction due to poor circulation to the genitalia.

I have found that I think more clearly and I am slightly more alert and talkative when I take ginkgo. However, I do not notice any significant effect on libido or erections as a result of using ginkgo.

Ginkgo is widely available in a variety of dosages and combinations, most commonly in 40 or 60 mg pills or capsules. The majority of the studies done thus far, on ginkgo as a treatment for dementia, have used daily dosages of 120 mg (50:1 concentration, 24% flavonoids).

Ginkgo is best taken early in the day, and no later than dinner. Few serious side effects have been noted in formal studies with ginkgo. In rare cases, mild stomach or intestinal complaints, headache, and allergic skin reactions have been mentioned, along with internal bleeding when ginkgo was combined with blood thinners such as aspirin or coumadin. It is best to make your physician aware that you are taking ginkgo if you are also taking prescribed medicines.

Ginkgo is not a true aphrodisiac in the sense that most users do not notice a clear or immediate sex-boosting effect. However, the long-term use of ginkgo may help with sexual dysfunction if the problem is due to poor circulation. The jury is still out as to whether ginkgo helps with antidepressant-induced sexual dysfunction.

SUMA

Suma (*Pfaffia paniculata*) is the dried root of a ground vine that grows in the tropical rain forests of South America. The root of suma contains saponins, including a group of novel chemicals called pfaffosides, as well as glycosides, phytoestrogens, nortriperpenes, and beta-ecdysones. It was introduced to this country as "Brazilian Ginseng" in order to capitalize on ginseng's reputation. This is misleading since the two herbs are not related in any way. Suma is known as *Para Toda* which means "for all things," since the indigenous peoples of the Amazon region have used the root of suma for generations as an energy and rejuvenating tonic, as well as a general cure-all for many types of illnesses. Suma has also been used as an aphrodisiac.

Human studies with suma have not been published in the Western medical literature. However, a rodent study provides a hint that suma does have some sex-boosting potential. Sexually potent and sexually sluggish, or impotent, male rats were treated orally with different amounts of damiana and suma fluid extracts. While having no effect on the copulatory behavior of sexually potent rats, both of the plant extracts—singly and in combination—improved the copulatory performance of impotent rats.

I have tried suma only once. I took four capsules, each containing 500 mg for a total of 2 g, on an empty stomach before breakfast. Within a short period of time, I felt a mild nausea that lasted an hour. I then noticed a light enhancement in visual clarity. I continued taking two capsules before breakfast and two before lunch daily for a few days. I experienced no nausea as a result of taking this lower dose. By the fourth day, I noticed a slight increase in energy and perhaps a slight increase in ease of erection, but the effects were subtle and I could not be certain. I also noticed that the type of energy I had was not necessarily that of a harsh stimulant type, but more of a calming and relaxed sense of well-being.

Suma ingestion has not been associated with any serious adverse reactions. However, comprehensive safety studies have not been undertaken, therefore much is unknown about the risks of daily intake for prolonged periods.

The optimum daily dosage of suma has not been established with any certainty. In my limited experience, total daily dosage can range from 1 to 2 g a day, with half taken in the morning and the other half with lunch. Suma, used by itself, appears to produce a subtle but pleasant tonic effect with no immediate significant influence on libido. Suma is best suited as a companion to other herbs such as muira puama and catuaba. Therefore, you may consider taking 500 mg or 1,000 mg of suma in addition to these herbs. Individuals who tend to notice the subtle effects of plant supplements may like suma. I have patients who are very sensitive to supplements and herbs, while others need to be hit by a massive dose of a powerful hormone to notice anything. Those who need a strong jolt to notice an effect will probably not appreciate the subtleties of suma.

ZALLOUH

Zallouh is made from the dried root of the herb *Ferula hermonis*, which grows at a height of about 2,000 meters above sea level on the side of Mount Hermoun between Lebanon and Syria. Zallouh has been used historically in the region as an aphrodisiac and stimulant, but only recently have scientists evaluated its chemical properties. Zallouh contains a number of compounds including ferulic acid and sesquiterpenes.

The crude oil from zallouh can enhance erectile function in rodents, however zallouh becomes toxic if used for a long period of time in high doses. In mice, the ingestion of 3 mg per kilogram of body weight of aqueous extract of zallouh for six weeks inhibited social aggression. Body weight and other sex accessory organ weights (such as that of the prostate and seminal vesicles) were significantly reduced. The ingestion of high doses of zallouh by male mice resulted in a significant reduction of their fertility.

There have been reports in lay magazine articles that human trials have been done in Lebanon at the Lebanese Center for Urology. Apparently, zallouh increased sexual desire and enhanced sexual performance in the subjects, but these studies have not yet been published on Medline. Since rodent studies indicate that high doses for prolonged periods may be toxic, it is best to take breaks from use until long-term human studies are published.

Traditionally, the roots of zallouh are made into a tea or eaten after being soaked in wine. Products are now available that have about 300 to 400 mg of dried root powder per capsule. I have not yet tried zallouh, so I do not have any personal insights regarding this herb.

I would not be surprised if there are hundreds of undiscovered natural substances that have a positive influence on the human sexual response. The ones that I have mentioned in this book are those known by our Western culture. I believe, with time, we will uncover additional herbs that have sex-boosting properties. Nature holds a treasure of secrets for us, and it is quite exciting to envision the possibilities in sexual enhancement just waiting to emerge.

Conclusion

Choosing the Sex Booster for You

With so many natural sex boosters readily available, how do you decide which ones are most appropriate for you? In this chapter, I provide suggestions to help you steer through this maze.

Several factors may influence your decision on which sex booster to choose. These factors include age; sex; health; body weight; medical conditions that you may have; concurrent use of prescription medicines; and your preference for herbs, supplements, or hormones. Furthermore, your choice depends on whether you have an interest in a fast-acting aphrodisiac or if you prefer a slower approach with increasing effects over several days; and, whether you prefer to boost libido or just enhance and prolong an erection or genital engorgement.

SEX BOOSTERS IN YOUTH

Generally, most people in their 20s and 30s are not necessarily looking to enhance their libido. If you are young, perhaps a raging libido is actually a hindrance, distracting you from studying at school or focusing on your career. Maybe the problem is premature ejaculation, or the anxiety of being with a new partner. Or, perhaps long hours spent at work or school have taken a toll on your mental health, and your sex drive has diminished. Another possibility is that the many years that you have spent with your partner or spouse has diminished the wonderful sexual relationship you once enjoyed. Fortunately, you're in luck. The proper use of natural sex boosters could well revive your lagging sex life.

SEX BOOSTERS IN MATURITY

As we age, a number of factors interfere with our ability to have a passionate sexual life. Hormone levels may drop; our physical endurance may decrease; we may become bored with our partner; we may be exposed to multiple stresses including financial, emotional, and problems with family life; and most commonly, there may be medical problems or certain medicines that we are taking that may interfere with libido or performance. Any older person with problems in his or her sex life should first have a consultation with a physician to make sure there are no medical reasons that would account for the waning sexuality. Also, it is particularly difficult to judge the ideal dosage of an herb or a combination of herbs that would be an effective treatment for seniors. Natural sex boosters can certainly help improve the mature person's sexual experiences, but it is recommended that older individuals start sex boosters in low dosages, and do so under medical supervision.

A FEW WORDS OF CAUTION

It is very important to be careful when taking certain sex supplements since some of them may interfere with a particular medical condition or with a prescription medicine. This applies to all ages, but especially to those people who are older. I recommend consulting with your health care provider before you take sex boosters—particularly yohimbe and the hormones DHEA, pregnenolone, and androstenedione.

Please note that it is very difficult to recommend dosages that would be appropriate for everyone reading this book. If you are the type of person who notices effects from taking small amounts of products, or you are sensitive to medicines and supplements, then start on the low end of the dosage suggestions. Depending on how a particular herb or supplement makes you feel, start with a low dose and gradually increase the dosage until you achieve the desired effect.

FAST-ACTING SEX BOOSTERS

I have come across many skeptics who doubt that natural sex boost-ers are effective. Well, the only thing these people have to do to be convinced is to take one of these speedy libido lifts, and they will soon be total converts. However, do not expect these natural prod-ucts to be as powerful as Viagra, Levitra, or the other newer drugs, in terms of their influence solely on erections. Natural sex boosters work a little slower, and are not as consistent as pharmaceuticals in causing erections or genital engorgement—although they often pro-vide additional benefits such as a libido boost or an enhancement in sensation that Viagra will not do.

Yohimbe is a consistently effective, quick-acting sex booster. It works within one or two hours after ingestion. The effects include enhanced sensation, clitoral engorgement, and longer-lasting erec-tions. Generally, both men and women find yohimbe to be on their top five list of sex boosters. The optimum dosage ranges from 100 mg to 300 mg. The drawback with yohimbe is that a high dose causes increased body heat, sweating, and a feeling of heart pound-ing. Sometimes it is tricky to find just the right dose that enhances genital swelling yet minimizes the side effects. The best way to find the ideal dosage for you is to start with 100 mg and gradually build up until the positive effects are maximized, yet the side effects do not distract from the sexual experience.

CDP-choline is another effective sex booster. At a dose of 500 mg to 750 mg, the effects are noticed within two to three hours of ingestion. Most people report enhanced sexual interest and better erections. Choline works well, too, at a similar dosage.

DMG, taken sublingually at a dose of 500 mg, increases skin sensation and interest in sex. The benefits are often noticed within hours, but are enhanced after two or three days of taking 250 to 500 mg twice daily—morning and midday. TMG, at a dose of 500 mg to 1,000 mg, also works within hours, but the full effects are noticed a day or two later.

NADH, at a dose of 5 to 10 mg, enhances sexual pleasure when taken on an empty stomach, with a mild effect on erection. The effects may be noticed within hours, yet may still be present the next day. A sublingual pill is available that dissolves in the mouth.

Androstenedione, at 25 mg to 50 mg, may work within an hour or two, but for others it may take from several hours to two or three days. Andro enhances libido and also has a mild positive effect on erections.

DHEA, taken in a dose of 25 mg or higher, may boost sexual interest within a few hours, and continues to be effective on the following day.

Tongkat ali is a reliable sex herb, which may start working within several hours on a high dose of 1,000 mg of the powder or 60 mg or more of the 100:1 extract. I personally prefer tongkat ali be taken in the morning in anticipation for sexual activity later in the afternoon or evening or for even the next day. Many patients report that high doses cause a feeling of restlessness and insomnia.

BOOSTING LIBIDO SLOWLY
BUT SURELY WITH HERBS

There are quite a number of nutrients, herbs, and hormones that boost libido and sexual pleasure over several days of use. Pick one of the following supplements and try it for a period of a week or two. Once you get a good feel for it, take a break for a few days, and then either return to it if you like it, or try another herb or supplement. If you plan to combine two herbs or nutrients, it may be a good idea to reduce the dose of each by about half.

Ashwagandha sometimes works within hours on the first day, but the effects are enhanced the second or third day of use. A dose of 1 to 2 g is effective for most people.

Catuaba, at a dose of 500 to 1,000 mg, taken once or twice daily, works mostly for erection or genital engorgement. The effects are best noticed by the third or fourth day of use.

Ginseng extract, at a dose of 100 mg or 200 mg, should produce results within a few days when taken daily in the morning.

Horny goat weed works well, and the effects are noticed on the third or fourth day of use. The suggested dose is 1 or 2 g daily.

Maca, at a dose of 1 to 3 g, taken daily in the morning, should enhance libido within a week. You may also notice an enhancement in energy and a slight improvement in mood.

Muira puama, at 0.5 g to 1.5 g, taken daily in the morning, produces a sex-boosting effect either on the first day, or within two to three days of use. Most of my patients report MP gives them a sense of well-being.

Tribulus may work the first day of use, but often the effects are more pronounced after the second or third day. A dose of 1 to 3 g may be taken for several days.

BOOSTING LIBIDO SLOWLY BUT SURELY WITH NUTRIENTS

There are several nutrients that I mentioned earlier in this chapter that could work well within hours of use on a high dose. These same nutrients may also be taken at a lower dosage for several days, and could provide a gradual libido enhancement—with fewer side effects.

CDP-choline may be taken at a dose of 250 mg once daily, such as before breakfast or lunch. Most people report enhanced sexual interest and better erections within a couple of days. Choline works well, too, at a similar dosage.

DMG, taken at a dose of 250 mg, enhances sensation, desire, and sexual performance. The benefits are often noticed within hours, but are increased after taking 250 mg twice a day, morning and midday, for two or three days. TMG, at a dose of 250 mg, may be taken each morning with results expected one, two, or three days later.

NADH, in a dosage of 2.5 mg or 5 mg, heightens sexual pleasure when taken on an empty stomach in the morning. The effects may be noticed within hours, yet are enhanced following several days of use.

Each fish oil capsule usually contains about 300 mg of a combination DHA and EPA. Take five capsules a day before or with breakfast for a week or two. The sex-enhancing effect of fish oils usually takes several days to notice. For a quicker effect, you may need to take six to ten capsules per day. However, be cautious when taking this many capsules; if you have a bleeding problem or are taking coumadin, aspirin, or other blood thinners, fish oils will increase the problem of thinning blood.

BOOSTING LIBIDO SLOWLY BUT SURELY WITH HORMONES

Three chapters in this book deal with the hormones androstene-dione, DHEA, and pregnenolone. As I have mentioned, these hormones are powerful sex boosters—but they also have side effects if misused or taken for prolonged periods. I strongly recommend you consult with a health care provider before using them.

Androstenedione or DHEA, at a dose of 10 mg to 25 mg, may be taken once daily in the morning or at lunch, for a maximum of three to five days per month. You should notice an effect within two to three days of use. By taking a long break from use, you would minimize any potential harm from using these powerful hormones.

Pregnenolone may be taken at a dose of 5 mg to 20 mg daily for a maximum of three to five days per month. Benefits are usually noticed by the third or fourth day.

SOLUTIONS FOR HIGH ANXIETY OR TENSION

The stress or anxiety of being with a new partner can certainly make it more difficult for men to get an erection or, for women, to be relaxed enough to get in the mood. There are several supplements that are helpful in this situation.

If you normally have a high libido and easily achieve erections but are just tense, kava—the root of a tree grown in the Pacific islands—can be a great help to you. Take one capsule containing 70 to 100 mg of kavalactones about two to fours hours before meeting your partner, or before intimacy. You'll be in a better mood, peaceful, and generally relaxed.

If you suffer from anxiety along with a reduced libido, the Ayurvedic herb ashwagandha is a good sex booster. Ashwagandha helps you relax, and at the same time has the potential to slightly increase your sexual interest. A dose of 500 to 1000 mg is often sufficient to achieve these positive results.

You may need to experiment with the dose and timing of kava and ashwagandha to find out the schedule and combination that works best for you. It is very difficult to recommend a dose that would be appropriate for everyone. For best results, some individuals may need to take kava or ashwagandha for a couple of days before planned sexual activity.

SOLUTIONS FOR PREMATURE EJACULATION

You barely get started and it's over. What do you do now? Reach for the remote control and turn on ESPN? Not a good idea if you want the relationship to continue.

If you ejaculate too soon, consider taking the nutrient 5-HTP. The substance 5-HTP stands for 5-hydroxytryptophan. This nutrient is absorbed into the bloodstream, and then travels to the brain where it converts into serotonin. If it is taken on an empty stomach, you may notice a feeling of relaxation within an hour. As I mentioned in Chapter 1, serotonin has an inhibitory effect on sex and ejaculation. A recommended dose for preventing premature ejaculation is 50 mg of 5-HTP taken about an hour or so before intercourse. Another option is to take 25 mg or 50 mg two or three times during the day before the planned evening sexual activity.

I have discussed many herbs and nutrients in this book that I believe have aphrodisiac properties and that work for me. These are just my personal preferences thus far, and this list may change as I experiment with various dosages of other herbs and nutrients for longer periods. Over time, various extracts and concentrations of these substances may become available that could very well be more effective and potent. As you try different herbs and nutrients, you will develop your own preference list.

As you can see, there are quite a number of supplements that are potential sex boosters. These natural aphrodisiacs offer a world of possibilities for enhancing your sex life. Since each of you reading this book has a different biochemistry, it is nearly impossible to recommend a fixed dosage regimen that would be appropriate for everyone. You may wish to try various products at different times and in different dosages until you find some that work for you. I find it quite pleasurable to experiment and try different sex boosters to see how they make me feel. I hope you will also take the opportunity to enjoy these interesting aphrodisiacs, and hope they help enhance your sexual pleasure and improve your love life! I am also quite certain that there are many natural aphrodisiacs, herbs, and compounds deep in woods or jungles that have not yet been discovered by modern medical science. I look forward to continuing my explorations into the fascinating field of natural sex boosters.

References

Androstenedione

Ballantyne, C.S., S.M. Phillips, J.R. MacDonald, et al. "The acute effects of androstenedione supplementation in healthy young males." *Can J Appl Physiol*, Vol. 25 (2000), pp. 68-78.

Brown, G.A., M.D. Vukovich, E.R. Martini, et al. "Endocrine responses to chronic androstenedione intake in 30- to 56-year-old men." *J Clin Endocrinol Metab*, Vol. 85 (2000), pp. 4074-4080.

Kachhi, P.N., and S.O. Henderson. "Priapism after androstenedione intake for athletic performance enhancement." *Ann Emerg Med*, Vol. 35 (2000), pp. 391-393.

Leder, BZ, et al. "Effects of oral androstenedione administration on serum testosterone and estradiol levels in postmenopausal women." *J Clin Endocrinol Metab*, Vol. 87 (Dec. 2002), No. 12, pp. 5449–5454.

Arginine

Chen, J, et al. "Effect of oral administration of high-dose nitric oxide donor L-arginine in men with organic erectile dysfunction: results of a double-blind, randomized, placebo-controlled study." *British Journal of Urology International*, Vol. 83 (Feb. 1999), No. 3, pp. 269–273.

Ito, T.Y., and A.S. Trant. "A double-blind placebo-controlled study of ArginMax, a nutritional supplement for enhancement of female sexual function." *J Sex Marital Ther*, Vol. 27 (Oct.-Dec. 2001), No.5, pp. 541–549.

Lebret, T, et al. "Efficacy and safety of a novel combination of L-arginine glutamate and yohimbine hydrochloride: a new oral therapy for erectile dysfunction." *European Urology*, Vol. 41 (Jun. 2002), No. 6, pp. 608–613.

Meston, C.M., and M. Worcel. "Effects of yohimbine plus L-arginine glutamate on sexual arousal in postmenopausal women with sexual arousal disorder." *Arch Sexual Behavior*,Vol. 31 (Aug. 2002), No. 4, pp. 323–332.

Ashwagandha

Abou-Douh, A.M. "New withanolides and other constituents from the fruit of Withania somnifera." *Arch Pharm*, Vol. 335 (Jun. 2002), No. 6, pp. 267–276.

Archana, R., and A. Namasivayam. "Antistressor effect of Withania somnifera." *J Ethnopharmacol*, Vol. 64 (Jan. 1999), No. 1, pp. 91–93.

Bhattacharya, S.K., et al. "Anxiolytic-antidepressant activity of Withania somnifera glycowithanolides: an experimental study." *Phytomedicine*, Vol. 7 (Dec. 2000), No. 6, pp. 463–469.

Dhuley, J.N. "Nootropic-like effect of ashwagandha (Withania somnifera L.) in mice." *Phytother Res*, Vol. 15 (Sept. 2001), No. 6, pp. 524–528.

Panda, S., and A. Kar. "Evidence for free radical scavenging activity of Ashwagandha root powder in mice." *Indian J Physiol Pharmacol*, Vol. 41 (Oct. 1997), No. 4, pp. 424–426.

Schliebs, R., et al. "Systemic administration of defined extracts from Withania somnifera (Indian Ginseng) and Shilajit differentially affects cholinergic but not glutamatergic and GABAergic markers in rat brain." *Neurochem Int*, Vol. 30 (Feb. 1997), No. 2, pp. 181–190.

Catuaba

Manabe, H., et al. "Effects of Catuaba extracts on microbial and HIV infection." *In Vivo*, Vol. 6 (Mar.-Apr. 1992), No. 2, pp. 161–165.

Choline and CDP-choline

Adibhatla, R.M. "Citicoline mechanisms and clinical efficacy in cerebral ischemia." *J Neurosci Res*, Vol. 70 (Oct. 2002), No. 2, pp. 133–139.

Adibhatla, R.M., et al. "Citicoline: neuroprotective mechanisms in cerebral ischemia." *J Neurochem*, Vol. 80 (Jan. 2002), No. 1, pp. 12–23.

Alvarez, X.A., et al. "Double-blind placebo-controlled study with citicoline in Alzheimer's disease patients. Effects on cognitive performance, brain bioelectrical activity and cerebral perfusion." *Methods Find Exp Clin Pharmacol*, Vol. 21 (Nov. 1999), No. 9, pp. 633–644.

Babb, S.M., et al. "Chronic citicoline increases phosphodiesters in the brains of healthy older subjects: an in vivo phosphorus magnetic resonance spectroscopy study." *Psychopharmacology (Berl)*, Vol. 161 (May 2002), No. 3, pp. 248–254.

Campos, E.C., et al. "Effect of citicoline on visual acuity in amblyopia: preliminary results." *Graefes Arch Clin Exp Ophthalmol*, Vol. 233 (May 1995), No. 5, pp. 307–312.

Lopez, G., I. Coviella, et al. "Effects of orally administered cytidine 5'-diphosphate choline on brain phospholipid content." *J Nutr Biochem*, Vol. 3 (Jun. 1992), No. 6, pp. 313–315.

Oshitari, T., et al. "Citicoline has a protective effect on damaged retinal ganglion cells in mouse culture retina." *Neuroreport*, Vol. 13 (Nov. 2002), No. 16, pp. 2109–2111.

Rejdak, R., et al. "Citicoline treatment increases retinal dopamine content in rabbits." *Ophthalmic Res*, Vol. 34 (May-Jun. 2002), No. 3, pp.146–149.

Wurtman, R.J., et al. "Effect of oral CDP-choline on plasma choline and uridine levels in humans." *Biochem Pharmacol*, Vol. 60 (2000), No. 7, pp. 989–992.

Cnidium Monnieri

Chiou, W.F., Y.L. Huang, C.F. Chen, and C.C. Chen. "Vasorelaxing effect of coumarins from Cnidium monnieri on rabbit corpus cavernosum." *Planta Med*, Vol. 67 (Apr. 2001), No.3, pp. 282–284.

Yang, L.L., M.C. Wang, L.G. Chen, and C.C. Wang. "Cytotoxic Activity of Coumarins from the Fruits of Cnidium monnieri on Leukemia Cell Lines." *Planta Med*, Vol. 69 (Dec. 2003), No. 12, pp. 1091–1095.

Damiana

Arletti, R., et al. "Stimulating property of Turnera diffusa and Pfaffia paniculata extracts on the sexual-behavior of male rats." *Psychopharmacology (Berl)*, Vol. 143 (Mar. 1999), No. 1, pp. 15–19.

Deer Antler Velvet

Allen, M., et al. "Elk velvet antler in rheumatoid arthritis: phase II trial." *Biol Res Nurs*, Vol. 3 (Jan. 2002), No. 3, pp. 111–118.

Conaglen, H.M., Suttie, J.M., and Conaglen, J.V. "Effect of deer velvet on sexual function in men and their partners: a double-blind, placebo-controlled study." *Arch Sex Behav*, Vol. 32 (Jun. 2003), No. 3, pp. 271–278.

Kropotov, A.V., et al. "Seasonal features of the effect of adaptogens on sex behavior of experimental animals." *Eksp Klin Farmakol*, Vol. 64 (Nov.-Dec. 2001), No. 6, pp. 60–62.

Zhang, H., et al. "Toxicological evaluation of New Zealand deer velvet powder. Part I: acute and subchronic oral toxicity studies in rats." *Food Chem Toxicol*, Vol. 38 (Nov. 2000), No. 11, pp. 985–90.

DHEA

Arlt, W, et al. "Dehydroepiandrosterone supplementation in healthy men with an age-related decline of dehydroepiandrosterone secretion." *J Clin Endocrinol Metab*, Vol. 86 (Oct. 2001), No. 10, pp. 4686–4692.

Hackbert, L., and J.R. Heiman. "Acute dehydroepiandrosterone (DHEA) effects on sexual arousal in postmenopausal women." *J Womens Health Gend Based Med*, Vol. 11 (Mar. 2002), No. 2, pp. 155–162.

Johannsson, G, et al. "Low dose dehydroepiandrosterone affects behavior in hypopituitary androgen-deficient women: a placebo-controlled trial." *J Clin Endocrinol Metab*, Vol. 87 (May 2002), No. 5, pp. 2046–2052.

Reiter, W.J., et al. "Dehydroepiandrosterone in the treatment of erectile dysfunction in patients with different organic etiologies." *Urol Res,* Vol. 29 (Aug. 2001), No. 4, pp. 278–281.

DMG

Niculescu, M.D., and S.H. Zeisel. "Diet, methyl donors and DNA methylation: interactions between dietary folate, methionine and choline." *J Nutr,* Vol. 132 (Aug. 2002), No. 8, pp. 2333S-2335S.

Fish Oils

Hirafuji, M., et al. "Docosahexaenoic acid potentiates interleukin-1beta induction of nitric oxide synthase through mechanism involving p44/42 MAPK activation in rat vascular smooth muscle cells." *Br J Pharmacol,* Vol. 136 (Jun. 2002), No. 4, pp. 613–619.

Peet, M., and D.F. Horrobin. "A dose-ranging study of the effects of ethyl-eicosapentaenoate in patients with ongoing depression despite apparently adequate treatment with standard drugs." *Arch Gen Psychiatry,* Vol. 59 (Oct. 2002), No. 10, pp. 913–919.

Rooke, J.A., et al. "Effects of feeding tuna oil on the lipid composition of pig spermatozoa and in vitro characteristics of semen." *Reproduction,* Vol. 121 (Feb. 2001), No. 2, pp. 315–322.

Segarra, A.B., et al. "Effects of dietary supplementation with fish oil, lard, or coconut oil on oxytocinase activity in the testis of mice." *Arch Androl,* Vol. 48 (May-Jun. 2002), No. 3, pp. 233–236.

Ginkgo

Ashton, A.K., et al. "Antidepressant-induced sexual dysfunction and Ginkgo Biloba." *Am J Psychiatry,* Vol. 157 (May 2000), No. 5, pp. 836–837.

Fies, P., and A. Dienel. "Ginkgo extract in impaired vision—treatment with special extract EGb 761 of impaired vision due to dry senile macular degeneration." *Wien Med Woch,* Vol. 152 (2002), No. 15–16, pp. 423–426.

Kang, B.J., et al. "A placebo-controlled, double-blind trial of Ginkgo biloba for antidepressant-induced sexual dysfunction." *Hum Psychopharmacol,* Vol. 17 (Aug. 2002), No. 6, pp. 279–284.

Ginseng

Gillis, C.N. "Panax ginseng pharmacology: a nitric oxide link?" *Biochem Pharmacol,* Vol. 54 (Jul 1997), No. 1, pp. 1–8.

Hong, B., et al. "A double-blind crossover study evaluating the efficacy of korean red ginseng in patients with erectile dysfunction: a preliminary report." *The Journal of Urology,* Vol. 168 (2002), pp. 2070–2073.

Murphy, L.L., and T.J. Lee. "Ginseng, sex behavior, and nitric oxide." *Ann NY Acad Sci,* Vol. 962 (May 2002), pp. 372–377.

Maca

Cicero, A.F., et al. "Hexanic Maca extract improves rat sexual performance more effectively than methanolic and chloroformic Maca extracts." *Andrologia,* Vol. 34 (Jun. 2002), No. 3, pp. 177–179.

Dini, A. et al. "Chemical composition of Lepidium meyenii." *Food Chem,* Vol. 49 (1994), pp. 347–349.

Gonzales, G.F., et al. "Effect of Lepidium meyenii (Maca), a root with aphrodisiac and fertility-enhancing properties, on serum reproductive hormone levels in adult healthy men." *J Endocrinol,* Vol. 176 (Jan. 2003), No. 1, pp. 163–168.

Gonzales, G.F., et al. "Lepidium meyenii (Maca) improved semen parameters in adult men."*Asian J Androl,* Vol. 3 (Dec. 2001), No. 4, pp. 301–303.

Piacente, S., et al. "Investigation of the tuber constituents of maca (Lepidium meyenii Walp.)." *J Agric Food Chem,* Vol. 50 (Sept. 2002), No. 20, pp. 5621–5625.

Muira Puama

Antunes, E., et al. "The relaxation of isolated rabbit corpus cavernosum by the herbal medicine Catuama and its constituents." *Phytother Res,* Vol. 15 (Aug. 2001), No. 5, pp. 416–421.

Da Silva, A.L., et al. "Anxiogenic properties of Ptychopetalum olacoides Benth. (Marapuama)." *Phytother Res,* Vol. 16 (May 2002), No. 3, pp. 223–226.

Waynberg, J., and S. Brewer. "Effects of Herbal vX on libido and sexual activity in premenopausal and postmenopausal women." *Adv Ther,* Vol. 17 (Sep.-Oct. 2000), No. 5, pp. 255–262.

Waynberg, J. 1990. "Aphrodisiacs: Contributions to the clinical validation of the traditional use of Psychopetalum guyanna." Presented at The First International Congress on Ethnopharmacology, 5–9 June, at Strasbourg, France.

NADH

Forsyth, L.M., et al. "Therapeutic effects of oral NADH on the symptoms of patients with chronic fatigue syndrome." *Ann Allergy Asthma Immunol,* Vol. 82 (Feb. 1999), No. 2, pp. 185–191.

Pregnenolone

Darnaudery, M., et al. "The neurosteroid pregnenolone sulfate infused into the medial septum nucleus increases hippocampal acetylcholine and spatial memory in rats." *Brain Res,* Vol. 951 (Oct. 2002), No. 2, pp. 237–242.

Mayo, W. "Pregnenolone sulfate and aging of cognitive functions: behavioral, neurochemical, and morphological investigations." *Horm Behav,* Vol. 40 (Sep. 2001), No. 2, pp. 215–217.

Suma

Arletti, R., et al. "Stimulating property of Turnera diffusa and Pfaffia paniculata extracts on the sexual-behavior of male rats." *Psychopharmacology (Berl),* Vol. 143 (Mar. 1999), No. 1, pp. 15–19

Balla, S.K. "Hydration of sickle erythrocytes using a herbal extract (Pfaffia paniculata) in vitro." *Br J Haemat,* Vol. 111 (Oct. 2000), No. 1, pp. 359–362.

Tongkat Ali

Ang, H.H., and T.H. Ngai. "Aphrodisiac evaluation in non-copulator male rats after chronic administration of Eurycoma longifolia Jack." *Fundam Clin Pharmacol,* Vol. 15 (Aug. 2001), No. 4, pp. 265–268.

Ang, H.H., and K.L. Lee. "Effect of Eurycoma longifolia Jack on libido in middle-aged male rats." *J Basic Clin Physiol Pharmacol,* Vol. 13 (2002), No. 3, pp. 249–254.

Ang, H.H, and M.K. Sim. "Eurycoma longifolia JACK and orientation activities in sexually experienced male rats." *Biol Pharm Bull,* Vol. 21 (Feb. 1998), No. 2, pp. 153–155.

Ang, H.H., T.H. Ngai, and T.H. Tan. "Effects of Eurycoma longifolia Jack on sexual qualities in middle aged male rats." *Phytomedicine,* Vol. 10 (2003), No. 6–7, pp. 590–593.

Tribulus

Adaikan, P.G., K. Gauthaman, and R.N. Prasad. *Ann Acad Med Singapore,* Vol. 29 (Jan. 2000), No. 1, pp. 22–26.

Antonio J., J. Uelmen, R. Rodriguez, and C. Earnest. "The effects of Tribulus terrestris on body composition and exercise performance in resistance-trained males." *Int J Sport Nutr Exerc Metab,* Vol. 10 (Jun. 2000), No. 2, pp. 208–15.

Bedir E., I.A. Khan, and L.A.Walker. "Biologically active steroidal glycosides from Tribulus terrestris." *Pharmazie,* Vol. 57 (Jul. 2002), No. 7, pp. 491–493.

De Combarieu, E., N. Fuzzati, M. Lovati, and E. Mercalli. "Furostanol saponins from Tribulus terrestris." *Fitoterapia,* Vol. 76 (Sep. 2003), No. 6, pp. 583–591.

Gauthaman K, A.P. Ganesan, and R.N. Prasad. "Sexual effects of puncturevine (Tribulus terrestris) extract (protodioscin): an evaluation using a rat model." *J Altern Complement Med.* Vol. 9 (Apr. 2003), No. 2, pp. 257–265.

Gauthaman, K., P.G. Adaikan, and R.N. Prasad. "Aphrodisiac properties of Tribulus Terrestris extract (Protodioscin) in normal and castrated rats." *Life Sci,* Vol. 71 (Aug. 2002), No. 12, pp. 1385–1396.

Huang, J.W., C.H. Tan, S.H. Jiang, and D.Y. Zhu. "Terrestrinins A and B, two new steroid saponins from Tribulus terrestris." *J Asian Nat Prod Res,* Vol. 5 (Dec. 2003), No. 4, pp. 285–290.

Wang, B., L. Ma, and T. Liu. "406 cases of angina pectoris in coronary heart disease treated with saponin of Tribulus terrestris." *Zhong Xi Yi Jie He Za Zhi,* Vol. 10 (Feb. 1990), No. 2, pp. 85–87.

Yohimbe

Lebret, T., et al. "Efficacy and safety of a novel combination of L-arginine glutamate and yohimbine hydrochloride: a new oral therapy for erectile dysfunction." *European Urology,* Vol. 41 (Jun. 2002), No. 6, pp. 608–613.

Meston, C.M., et al. "The effects of yohimbine plus L-arginine glutamate on sexual arousal in postmenopausal women with sexual arousal disorder." *Archives of Sexual Behavior,* Vol. 31 (Aug. 2002), No. 4, pp. 323–332.

Vogt, H.J., et al. "Double-blind, placebo-controlled safety and efficacy trial with yohimbine hydrochloride in the treatment of nonorganic erectile dysfunction." *International Journal of Impotence Research,* Vol. 9 (Sep. 1997), No. 3, pp. 155–161.

Zallouh

Hadidi, K.A., T. Aburjai, and A.K. Battah. "A comparative study of Ferula hermonis root extracts and sildenafil on copulatory behaviour of male rats." *Fitoterapia,* Vol. 74 (Apr. 2003), No. 3, pp. 242–246.

Khleifat, K., M.H. Homady, K.A. Tarawneh, and J. Shakhanbeh. "Effect of Ferula hormonis extract on social aggression, fertility and some physiological parameters in prepubertal male mice." *Endocr J,* Vol. 48 (Aug. 2001), No. 4, pp. 473–482.

El-Thaher T.S., K.Z. Matalka, H.A.Taha, and A.A. Badwan. "Ferula harmonis 'zallouh' and enhancing erectile function in rats: efficacy and toxicity study." *Int J Impot Res,* Vol. 13 (Aug. 2001), No. 4, pp. 247–251.

Visit
Dr. Ray Sahelian's
Website at

www.raysahelian.com

for further information about natural supplements and the nutritional approach to treating medical conditions.

Index

Acetylcholine, 13, 14, 16, 30, 37, 38, 39, 84

Aging-related problems, 19–23, 37–41, 43–47, 112

ALA. *See* Alpha-linolenic acid.

Alpha 2-adrenoceptors, 99

Alpha-1-adrenergic receptors, 15

Alpha-linolenic acid (ALA), 59

Andro. *See* Androstenedione.

Androgens, 19–20, 43, 44, 45, 56, 84

Androstenediol, 19

Androstenedione (andro), 19–23, 43, 44, 45, 84, 86
experiences with, 20–21
research on, 19–20
side effects of, 21–22, 23

Anxiety, help for, 29–30, 32, 116–117

Arginine, 15, 25–28, 98, 99
experiences with, 27

research on, 25–27
side effects of, 27

Ashwagandha, 29–32
experiences with, 30–31
research on, 29–30
side effects of, 31

Ayurveda, 29

Bantu, 97

Betaine. *See* TMG.

Bioflavonoids, 26

Brazil, 33, 34

Brazilian Ginseng. *See* Suma.

Catuaba, 33–35, 77
experiences with, 33–34
research on, 33
side effects of, 34

CDP-choline, 16, 37–41
experiences with, 39–40
research on, 38–39

side effects of, 40

cGMP. *See* Cyclic guanosine monophosphate.

Chemistry of sex, 13–17

Chinese ginseng. *See* Ginseng, Asian.

Choline, 16, 37–41, 49, 50, 52
  experiences with, 39–40
  research on, 38–39
  side effects of, 40

Citicoline. *See* CDP-choline.

Cnidium monnieri, 103–104

Corpora cavernosa, 14, 15, 16, 63, 76, 92, 93, 99, 104

Corynanthe yohimbe, 97

Cyclic guanosine monophosphate (cGMP), 15, 27

Cytidine 5'-diphosphocholine, 37

Damiana, 25, 104–105, 108

Deer antler velvet, 105–106

Dehydroepiandrosterone (DHEA), 19, 20, 22, 43–47, 84, 85, 86
  experiences with, 45–46
  research on, 44–45
  side effects of, 46

DHA. *See* Docosahexanoic acid.

DHEA. *See* Dehydroepiandrosterone.

DHT. *See* Dihydrotestosterone.

Dihydrotestosterone (DHT), 21, 43, 46

Dimethylgycine (DMG), 37, 49–53
  experiences with, 51
  research on, 49–50
  side effects of, 51–52

DMG. *See* Dimethylgycine.

Docosahexanoic acid (DHA), 55, 56, 57, 59

Dopamine, 14, 15–16, 38, 39, 50, 63, 80, 84, 99

Eicosapentanoic acid (EPA), 55, 56, 57, 59

Eleutherococcus Chinensis. See Ginseng, Siberian.

Endothelial cells, 15, 63, 93

EPA. *See* Eicosapentanoic acid.

Epimedium, 67

Epimedium brevicornum, 67

Epimedium koreanum, 67

Epimedium sagittatum (ES), 67, 68

Epinephrine, 14, 16, 17

Erectile dysfunction, 15, 16, 25, 26, 44–45, 61–62, 63, 97, 98

Erection, 14–15, 16, 17, 27, 39, 40, 45, 92, 99, 100

Erythroxylum catuaba, 33

ES. *See Epimedium sagittatum*.

Estrogen, 19, 20, 21, 43, 84

Ethyl-EPA, 56

Eurycoma longifolia jack, 87, 90
Exercise, 18

FDA, 23
Female Sexual Arousal
    Disorder, 99
Ferula hermonis, 109
Finasteride, 46
Fish oils, 18, 55–60
    experiences with, 57–58
    research on, 55–56
    side effects of, 58
5-HT. *See* 5-hydroxy-
    tryptamine.
5-HTP. *See* 5-hydroxy-
    tryptophan.
5-hydroxytryptamine (5-HT),
    17
5-hydroxytryptophan (5-HTP),
    17
Flaxseed oil, 59

GABA, 30
Ginkgo, 25, 75, 106–107
Ginseng, 15, 25, 61–65
    American, 61, 62
    Asian, 61, 63
    experiences with, 63–64
    research on, 61–62
    Siberian, 61
    side effects of, 64
Glutathione, 80
Glycine, 50
Guanylate cyclase, 15

Homocysteine, 50
Hormones, 112
    androstenedione, 19–23, 43,
        84, 86
    DHEA, 19, 22, 43–47, 84, 86
    pregnenolone, 19, 83–86
Horny goat weed, 67–69
    experiences with, 68
    research on, 67
    side effects of, 68
Hypopituitarism, 44

Icariin, 68, 69
ICP. *See* Intracavernous
    pressure.
Intracavernous pressure (ICP),
    92

Korean ginseng. *See* Ginseng,
    Asian.

L-arginine. *See* Arginine.
Lecithin, 16, 37
Lepidium meyenii, 71
Libido, enhancement of, 20,
    22, 25–26, 45–46, 75–77,
    80–81, 84–85, 87–88, 89, 90,
    93, 94, 97, 100
Long Jack. *See* Tongkat ali.

Maca, 71–73
    experiences with, 72
    research on, 71–72
    side effects of, 73

Marapuama. *See* Muira puama.

Materia Medica, 105

Methylation, 49

Methyl donor, 49, 50

MF. *See* Mounting frequency.

Mounting frequency (MF), 92

MP. *See* Muira puama.

Muira puama (MP), 34, 75–77

   experiences with, 76–77

   research on, 75–76

   side effects of, 77

Muirapuamine, 76

NADH. *See* Nicotinamide adenine dinucleotide.

Neurosteroid, 84

Neurotransmitters, 13–17, 84

Nicotinamide adenine dinucleotide (NADH), 16, 79–82

   experiences with, 80–81

   research on, 79–80

   side effects of, 81

Nitric oxide (NO), 13, 15, 20, 25, 27, 30, 56, 63, 68, 93

Nitric oxide synthase, 15, 30

NO. *See* Nitric oxide.

Nonalcoholic steatohepatitis, 50

Norandrostenedione, 19

Norepinephrine, 14, 15, 16–17, 50, 63, 99

Nutrition, 18

Omega-3 fatty acids, 55

Panax ginseng. See Ginseng, Asian.

Panax quinquefolius. See Ginseng, American.

Pantocrin, 105

Para Toda, 107

Pasak bumi. *See* Tongkat ali.

Pausinystalia yohimbe, 97

PC. *See* Phosphatidylcholine.

Pfaffia paniculata, 104

Phenylalanine, 16

Phosphatidylcholine (PC), 37, 38

Postmenopausal women, 26, 44, 98–99

Potency wood. *See* Muira puama.

Preg. *See* Pregnenolone.

Pregnenolone (Preg), 19, 20, 83–86

   experiences with, 84–85

   research on, 83

   side effects from, 85

Priapism, 22

Progesterone, 84

Prolactin, 63

Propranolol, 46

Protodioscin, 93

Prozac, 17, 106

Psychological-related problems, 26, 98, 102, 116–117

Ptychopetalum olacoides, 75

Puncture vine. *See* Tribulus terrestris.

Pycnogenol, 26

S-adenosylmethionine (SAMe), 49, 50, 52

SAMe. *See* S-adenosylmethionine.

Saponins, 62, 93, 107

Serotonin, 14, 17

Sexual dysfunction, in women, 25–26, 98–99

She Chuang Zi, 103

SSRI, 17, 106

Suma, 107–109

Testosterone, 19, 20, 43, 44, 45, 84

Tetramethylglycine. *See* Choline.

TMG. *See* Trimethylglycine.

Tongkat ali, 87–90
    experiences with, 88–89
    research on, 87–88
    side effects of, 90

Tribulus. *See* Tribulus terrestris.

Tribulus terrestris (TT), 91–95
    experiences with, 93–94
    research on, 91–92

side effects of, 94

Trimethylglycine (TMG), 37, 49–53
    experiences from using, 51
    research on, 50
    side effects of, 51–52

TT. *See* Tribulus terrestris.

Turnera aphrodisiaca, 104

Turnera diffusa, 104

Tyrosine, 16, 80

Vaginal photoplethysmograph, 99

Vaginal pulse amplitude, 26, 99

Viagra, 15, 97

Withania somniferum, 30

Withanolides, 30, 32

Yin Yang Huo, 67

Yohimbe, 15, 17, 97–102
    experiences with, 99–100
    research on. *See* Yohimbine, research on.
    side effects of, 100–101

Yohimbine, 15, 26, 97–99, 101, 102
    research on, 98–99

Zallouh, 109

About the Author

Ray Sahelian, MD, is a popular and respected physician and medical writer internationally recognized as a moderate voice in the evaluation of cutting-edge nutrients, herbs, and hormones. He has discussed the latest health and medical research on CNN and numerous national television programs including *Dateline NBC.* He has been cited by countless magazines including *Newsweek,* been quoted in hundreds of domestic and foreign newspapers, and reached millions of radio listeners nationwide.

Dr. Sahelian obtained a bachelor's degree in nutrition from Drexel University, and completed his doctoral training at Thomas Jefferson Medical School, both in Philadelphia. He is certified by the American Board of Family Practice. He is the best-selling author of more than a dozen books including *Mind Boosters* and *The Stevia Cookbook.* He currently resides in the Los Angeles area.

Dr. Sahelian's website, **www.RaySahelian.com,** contains extensive information on natural supplements and nutritional approaches to healing.

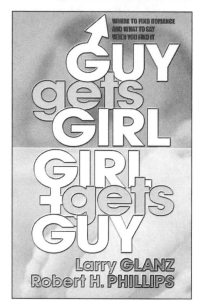

GUY GETS GIRL, GIRL GETS GUY

Where to Find Romance and What to Say When You Find It

Larry Glanz and Robert H. Phillips

Nobody said that meeting someone is easy. But the fact is that people begin romantic relationships every single day. The trick is to know how to go about it, and this is the book that will let you in on all the secrets and get you started in the right direction. *Guy Gets Girl, Girl Gets Guy* provides all the important basics, including how to successfully meet, greet, and—ultimately—win that special someone.

Guy Gets Girl, Girl Gets Guy takes a practical look at the wheres and how-tos of locating and attracting that one right person. Part One focuses on who you are and who you want to be. It offers proven suggestions for enhancing your "inner" and "outer" assets. It then helps you consider and select the qualities you would like to see in your future mate. Once you know who you are and who you would like to meet, the fun begins. Part Two provides a guide to the places you can go to meet new people—from the hottest websites to the trendiest night spots; from new and unusual places to common hangouts that are probably right under your nose.

This book even provides you with clever and effective ice breakers designed to launch your first conversation—a conversation that can lead to that first date, and maybe even a lifetime of love. With *Guy Gets Girl, Girl Gets Guy,* you have no more excuses to be lonely.

Larry Glanz is a relationships expert. He has spent over twenty years studying and analyzing mating customs in the United States. Based on this work, he has developed effective relationship strategies and techniques. He is the coauthor of *How to Start a Romantic Encounter.*

$13.95 US / $22.95 CAN • 208 pages • 6 x 9-inch paperback • ISBN 0-7570-0126-2

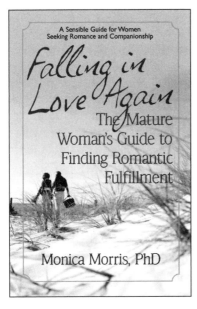

A Sensible Guide for Women
Seeking Romance and Companionship

Falling in
Love Again
The Mature
Woman's Guide to
Finding Romantic
Fulfillment

Monica Morris, PhD

FALLING IN LOVE AGAIN

The Mature Woman's Guide to Finding Romantic Fulfillment

Monica Morris, PhD

Like millions of women, social psychologist Dr. Monica Morris found herself unexpectedly single late in life. The road wasn't an easy one, but Dr. Morris found her way to a new love. In *Falling in Love Again,* Dr. Morris shares not only her experiences but also the knowledge she gained along the way, providing an empowering resource for mature women who are looking for romance and companionship.

The author begins by exploring your expectations of finding love, thus preparing you for the real world. She then looks at the need for self-assurance and poise, and offers numerous ways to bolster self-esteem. Dr. Morris then provides dozens of sensible suggestions for finding that special someone—from personal ads to online dating to matchmaking services. Included are important details about costs, accessibility, and precautions. Dr. Morris even addresses intimate questions regarding sex, living together, personal needs, and independence. Finally, she provides a unique resource of services, websites, and organizations designed to help you find a significant other—or to just have fun.

There is life after loneliness. Both compassionate and practical, *Falling in Love Again* is your guide to finding a new love and a new life.

Monica Morris received an MA and PhD in sociology from the University of Southern California. Her areas of expertise include social psychology, sociology of emotion, and medical sociology. She was a professor of sociology in the California State University System for over twenty years. A widely published author, Dr. Morris resides with her husband in southern California.

$14.95 US / $24.95 CAN • 224 pages • 6 x 9-inch paperback • ISBN 0-7570-0136-X

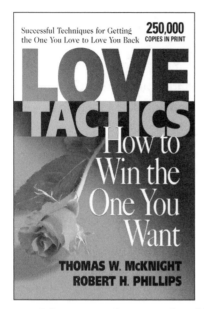

Successful Techniques for Getting the One You Love to Love You Back **250,000 COPIES IN PRINT**

THOMAS W. McKNIGHT
ROBERT H. PHILLIPS

LOVE TACTICS

How to Win the One You Want

Thomas McKnight and Robert H. Phillips

Maybe that very special someone is not as far out of reach as you think. Maybe what you need are a few effective strategies to finally make the right moves. Even if you're very shy, a little on the quiet side, or simply not the social success you'd like to be, *Love Tactics* may have the answers you've been looking for.

It's all here—how to build self-confidence, exhibit positive character traits, gain trust, and keep that special someone interested and hoping for a true commitment. *Love Tactics* will tell you all you need to know—from taking that first step and summoning up the courage to ask for a date, to sitting back and enjoying being with the one you want after you've won their heart!

Written in a warm, easy-going style, this book offers a wealth of practical advice on how to get the one you love to love you back. So don't just stand there—get out and stir up some hearts!

Thomas McKnight is a relationships expert. His columns on meeting the right person have appeared in leading U.S. singles newspapers and magazines over the past fifteen years. He has conducted dozens of relationship workshops throughout the country, and has also appeared on numerous radio and television shows, including Oprah.

Robert H. Phillips is a practicing psychologist and the director of the Center for Coping located in Westbury, New York. He is also the best-selling author of eight books dealing with various chronic health conditions, including *Coping With Lupus* and *Coping With Osteoarthritis*.

$12.95 US / $19.50 CAN • 208 pages • 6 x 9-inch paperback • ISBN 0-7570-0037-1